CRYSTALS FOR BEGINNERS

Unlock the Potential in Crystals for Healing and Energy

(Energy Protection Including Exact Rituals and Crystals to Harness Your Spirituality)

Carroll Chapin

Published by Harry Barnes

Carroll Chapin

All Rights Reserved

Crystals for Beginners: Unlock the Potential in Crystals for Healing and Energy (Energy Protection Including Exact Rituals and Crystals to Harness Your Spirituality)

ISBN 978-1-7751430-1-7

All rights reserved. No part of this guide may be reproduced in any form without permission in writing from the publisher except in the case of brief quotations embodied in critical articles or reviews.

Legal & Disclaimer

The information contained in this book is not designed to replace or take the place of any form of medicine or professional medical advice. The information in this book has been provided for educational and entertainment purposes only.

The information contained in this book has been compiled from sources deemed reliable, and it is accurate to the best of the Author's knowledge; however, the Author cannot guarantee its accuracy and validity and cannot be held liable for any errors or omissions. Changes are periodically made to this book. You must consult your doctor or get professional medical advice before using any of the suggested remedies, techniques, or information in this book.

Upon using the information contained in this book, you agree to hold harmless the Author from and against any damages, costs, and expenses, including any legal fees potentially resulting from the application of any of the information provided by this guide. This disclaimer applies to any damages or injury caused by the use and application, whether directly or indirectly, of any advice or information presented, whether for breach of contract, tort, negligence, personal injury, criminal intent, or under any other cause of action.

You agree to accept all risks of using the information presented inside this book. You need to consult a professional medical practitioner in order to ensure you are both able and healthy enough to participate in this program.

Table of Contents

INTRODUCTION 1

CHAPTER 1: WHAT ARE CRYSTALS? 5

CHAPTER 2: AN ABUNDANCE OF CRYSTALS 40

CHAPTER 3: HOW DO I USE CRYSTALS TO HEAL MYSELF? 47

CHAPTER 4: BEGINNING OF CRYSTAL HEALING 56

CHAPTER 5: HOW CRYSTAL HEALING WORKS 69

CHAPTER 6: THE WORLD OF CRYSTALS 72

CHAPTER 7: CHOOSING YOUR CRYSTALS 102

CHAPTER 8: CHOOSING THE RIGHT CRYSTAL 108

CHAPTER 9: HOW CRYSTALS AND CHAKRAS RELATE FOR YOUR WELLBEING 125

CHAPTER 10: HOW TO START A CRYSTAL COLLLECTION 130

CHAPTER 11: HOW TO CHOOSE YOUR CRYSTAL? 150

CHAPTER 12: OVERVIEW ON VISUALIZATION 162

CONCLUSION 181

Introduction

Healing with crystals goes back at least as far as Babylon and Ancient Egypt and it is believed that crystals have been valued and sought after since monolithic times, perhaps for their usefulness as tools with sharp cutting edges but perhaps their metaphysical properties were recognised even then. Throughout all of recorded history crystals and gemstones have been prized, revered, worshipped, bought and sold, shaped, polished, and have been used for everything from jewellery, ornaments, ceremonial burial items, religious relics, amulets and talismans, to tools of divination, magical devices and a cornucopia of medical elixirs and ointments, as well as for their healing effect on the mind, body and spirit. There are hundreds of different types of crystals out there and thousands of variants of these crystal types and each carries their own individual meanings, properties, and qualities in various degrees and strength. Birthstone connections

Ruling Planets

Zodiac associations

Energetic frequencies

Chakra connections

Making use of crystal energy on a daily basis gives access to a wealth of energy and information useful for all manner of trials and tribulations as well as celebrations. The body, mind, and spirit are intrinsically linked as one and if there is an imbalance in one it affects all three. The power of crystals is utilised by understanding and directing the energy contained within or emanating from the entire being of the crystal itself. Over thousands of years, through practice and error, methods have been discovered and developed that allow us as individuals to make the most of the power of crystals in order to support and aid our own wellbeing and the wellbeing of those around us. Many crystal's magical properties are extremely well known, and for thousands of years have held honoured positions within mystical rituals and ceremonial rites. Modern enthusiasts believe the true power of crystals lay in their ability to soothe and calm the emotions and redirect and maintain the flow of positive energy. The natural vibrational energies contained within crystals compliment and strengthen those of the human body and have been known to positively influence:

Self-expression and creativity

Vitality

Blood pressure

Blood sugar levels

Mood swings and depression

Sleeplessness and nightmares

Undue worry and stress

Headaches and migraines

Arthritis

General aches and pains

All manner of illnesses relating to the organs

Conditions affecting the ears, nose and throat

Choosing to bring the healing power of crystals into your life will begin a chain of actions leading to positive change and even a single visit with a professional Reiki healer with bring about instant and lasting results both psychically and emotionally, which ultimately leads to greater power and control over one's life and deep feelings of happiness and joy.

Chapter 1: What Are Crystals?

Before you can properly understand how crystals work and what they can do for you, it's important to understand what they are and where they come from. The minerals and formation processes can have an influence on the appearance and the abilities of crystals.

A Brief History of Crystals

Crystals have been a part of life since the dawn of our species, and records of the use of crystals can be dated all the way back to the ancient Sumerians. The Sumerians used crystals in almost all of their magic formulas. Bracelets with amber beads have been found in Britain that date back 10,000 years. Amber is not naturally found in England, meaning they have traveled long distances to get there. This shows us that amber was important enough to the people that they would carry these beads all the way with them.

The ancient Egyptians often used stones such as lapis lazuli, emerald, and clear quartz for their jewelry and commonly carved grave masks out of these gemstones.

The use of crystals and gemstones became especially popular in ancient Greece, and most of the crystal names we use today originate from this era. Even the word crystal comes from the Greek word krustallos meaning "ice". They used this word because the people believed that crystals were ice frozen so solidly that they would never melt. Different crystals were often associated with the gods and used in religious rituals and to decorate their temples. The Greeks also had many superstitions that involved crystals, such as wearing amethyst to avoid getting drunk or having a hangover or rubbing hematite (a crystal associated with Ares, the god of war) all over their bodies before battle believing it would make them invulnerable from then on.

Most religious texts such as the Koran and the Bible refer to crystals and gemstones several times, and many religious rituals incorporate crystals or assign a significant meaning to certain types of crystals. In many cultures, green stones were a symbol of life, and people were often buried with one of these stones over their heart.

The Chinese culture has always put special emphasis on jade, recognizing it as a kidney healing stone, and around 1,000 years ago, emperors were often buried in jade armor. Instruments in the form of chimes were commonly made and hung in homes and places of business, and even some of the characters in Chinese writing were designed to resemble jade beads.

Crystals no longer have such a deep cultural and significance as they used to, though they are still a powerful tool when it comes to healing and improving the lives of those who use them. Some of the symbolism connected with stones is still incorporated into modern culture in small ways, especially in books and films, such as a green stone being a core element of restoring life to a dying world or returning a broken-off shard to a magical crystal that keeps the world in balance. Crystals are also still a popular subject for scientists to study, and there are many scholarly courses and professional careers that concern the use of crystals and their abilities.

What Is a Crystal?

The term crystal or crystalline generally refers to a solid material in which clusters of atoms are arranged together in a regular geometric pattern, often resulting in prominent facets (though not always). By piling these clusters of atoms together in a repeating pattern, the crystal will grow larger. This pattern extends outward in three dimensions. Most crystals are rock formations, but there are some exceptions such as ice crystals and sugar. The type of pattern and structure of the atom cluster sets the type of crystal and is usually affected by how the crystal forms. The most common type of crystal found in everyday life is salt, and it can easily be used in experiments in growing crystals.

Gemstones

The term gemstone often comes to mind when talking about crystals, but there is a difference between a gemstone and a crystal. Gemstones are rare rock formations that can be used for decoration and jewelry and classified as precious or semi-precious, while crystals are structures of atoms arranged in a geometric pattern that extend into three dimensions. Most gemstones, such as diamonds, amber, and sapphire, are considered forms of crystal, but not all types of crystals are considered gemstones. Just as with crystals, gemstones can have a base construction of minerals or a more organic origin, as can be seen with amber. It can be especially important to know the difference between the two when buying crystals, as you might not be buying what you expect, and gemstones are usually more expensive than crystals.

How Do Crystals Form?

There are several ways by which crystals form. The general process is called crystallization. The most common form of crystallization is growing it from a liquid. As a liquid filled with minerals and other matter molecules condenses into gas form, the mineral molecules will remain solid and start packing themselves together in an attempt to remain stable, and a crystal is formed. The more the water condenses, the more molecules that will be packed together and the larger the crystal becomes. Not all molecules will form crystals, and the type of minerals present in the liquid will determine the color, density, shape, and type of crystal. If a solid structure is already present (i.e. a rock standing in a pool of mineral-rich water), the molecules will cling to it and the crystal formation will grow into this structure.

Another way crystals are formed is by cooling liquids. In much the same way, different types of molecules cluster together in a repeating pattern to form the crystals. The most common occurrence is molten lava cooling down, forming crystals within the rocks, which is one of the reasons why crystals are often abundant in areas with many volcanoes and tectonic plates nearby.

In some rare occasions, crystals can be formed by compressing gas into a solid form. This requires incredibly large amounts of pressure and usually takes hundreds of years to form a decently-sized crystal. Diamonds are formed by compressing carbon in this way, and it is because of the rarity of the right conditions and the amount of time it takes to form a diamond that makes them so incredibly expensive.

Outside factors such as general temperature, available space, available minerals, cooling speed, and humidity, as well as many other minor factors, will help determine the type of crystal that will form.

Where Do Crystals Come From?

Different crystals can be found in various regions due to the specific minerals and other elements available, but there are certain types of places where crystals tend to grow. Crystals generally form in rocky areas and under the ground, especially if these places remain undisturbed. Most of the earth's bedrock is one form of a crystal or another. As mentioned above, some crystals are formed within cooling lava, and this is where most of the world's crystals and gemstones are found. Lava comes from beneath the earth's crust and is sometimes pushed through to the surface, forming layers. The movement of the earth's tectonic plates have a similar effect, and this is how new crystals are created. Some crystals are formed immediately as the lava on the surface cools quickly, but others take much longer to form further down where the lava cools at a much slower pace. The speed at which a crystal is formed usually determines its size.

In some cases, the movement of the lava or earth creates empty spaces where water vapors are condensed into a mineral-rich liquid which will eventually grow into different crystals. Many underground caverns are damp and desolate enough that large clusters of crystals can grow for hundreds of years. Geodes form when gas or liquid is allowed to crystallize in a small cavity inside rocks and stones. Agate is a very common crystal to find inside geodes, and the majority of the world's geodes will have at least one or two layers of agate as a crust. In some cases, the cavity inside a geode will be completely filled with crystallized chalcedony and you will have a solid piece of agate, but it is also possible that you will have several layers of agate and another type of crystal, usually quartz, growing in the very center of the geode.

In some areas that have mineral-rich earth, it is possible to find small crystals scattered about or in the uppermost layer of the ground. The area will determine the types of crystals that can be found. Individual crystals are more likely than clusters, and many of these crystals will go unnoticed in their raw form. In some sandy areas, it is possible to find crystal formations such as desert roses and sand crystals. There are also a few places in the world where the sand consists of tiny crystals that are worn down. Quartz is an important mineral in sand formation, and it is often found that many sand grains are, in fact, quartz crystals.

There are also a few types of crystals that are grown from organic matter, such as amber, which is crystallized tree sap, or calcite and aragonite, which are produced by most mollusks.

Crystal Lattice

The term crystal lattice refers to the specific type of three-dimensional pattern in which the atoms are connected to form the crystal, and it can also be called the structure of the crystal. The lattice of a crystal is a key component in classifying crystals, as each type of crystal has a unique lattice. Many outside influences such as radiation, exposure to the elements, the way in which the crystal forms, and chemical impurities can affect the shape, color, and size of a crystal, but the lattice will remain the same. This is why two stones that look completely different from each other in color and shape can still be classified as the same type of crystal. The lattice will determine the number of faces (flat surfaces that form the shape of the crystal) a crystal has, as well as how they are placed in relation to each other.

As mentioned above, all crystals are formed through repeating geometric patterns, and there are seven specific types of patterns that occur. These types are lattice types. Crystal structures can be reduced to the smallest possible form of the pattern that can be repeated in three dimensions. This singular part of the lattice is called the unit cell, and it forms the base of the lattice used to create a crystal. A unit cell consists of a few atoms packed together in a set geometric shape which is repeated over and over again to form the lattice of the crystal. The three dimensions in which the pattern is repeated roughly indicate the different directions that the growth of the crystal takes place. The growth in the three dimensions is often represented by crystallographic axes, imaginary lines that intersect at 90-degree angles in the center of the crystal lattice. There are three axes used to represent the dimensions; they are simply referred to as the x-axis, y-axis, and z-axis, and they are usually perfectly perpendicular to each other. This set of axes is used frequently in science and math, but it also forms the core of 3D editing programs. In such programs, an object can be moved or altered forward and backward, to the left and right, and up and down, and each of these types of direction is indicated by an axis. The same concept is applied to a crystal lattice. The symmetry along each axis plays a large role in determining the type of lattice in a crystal.

Symmetry is an important element of crystal lattices. It refers to how the pattern is repeated, specifically how one cell unit is connected to the next. There are two different types of symmetry: translational symmetry and point symmetry. Translational symmetry is where the pattern is repeated simply through movement along a line or within a certain volume. As an example, if a cube-shaped cell unit is repeated by placing the units next to or on top of each other, translational symmetry is used to form a cubic lattice. Point symmetry is where the repetition occurs around a central point, such as in the cases of rotation, reflection, and inversion, along with others. An example of point symmetry is when a triangular unit cell is rotated around a central point in all three dimensions to form a triangle-based pyramid.

The initial shape of the cell unit and the type of symmetry determines the type of lattice that will be formed. Below we will go over the different types of crystal lattice in detail:

Isometric

This is also often called the cubic lattice, and it's built on a square-shaped cell unit. In this case, the crystallographic axes have perfect symmetry and are usually the same length. The axes can also often be applied diagonally and still be perfectly symmetrical. The different planes of the crystal that run parallel with each other will always be matched in shape and size. Cube- and diamond-shaped crystals are the most common results of this lattice type. Good examples of crystals with an isometric type lattice are magnetite and garnet.

Hexagonal

The hexagonal lattice system has a fourth axis. One axis runs vertically, but rather than two horizontal lines cutting each other to form four 90-degree corners, three lines meet each other to form three 120-degree corners. These three lines are no longer perpendicular to each other but are still perpendicular to the vertical line. The three 120-degree axes are usually symmetric and of equal length, while the fourth, perpendicular line can be longer or shorter. This lattice type results in crystals with eight faces, and crystals usually form prisms and pyramids with a six-sided base. The most common crystals with a hexagonal type lattice are high quartz, beryl, and apatite.

Tetragonal

Similar to the isometric system, this lattice system has three axes that meet in 90-degree corners. One of the axes, however, can be extended or shortened, forming a rectangular shape. Crystals with this type of lattice tend to have six faces, where the base and opposite face form a perfect square shape and the other four faces form rectangles. Some good examples of these types of crystals are cassiterite and zircon.

Rhombohedral

This system is similar to both the tetragonal system by having three perpendicular (meaning they all form 90-degree corners) axes, with one axis longer or shorter than the other two. It also has six faces, but rather than forming a perfectly square base, these crystals tend to form a base that is the shape of a diamond (also called a rhombus). Crystals with this type of lattice include low quartz, tourmaline, and dolomite.

Orthorhombic

This is another lattice system with three axes that meet perpendicularly, but unlike the other systems, none of the three axes are of the same length. These crystals tend to have six faces, but the base face forms an irregular four-sided shape that isn't a square, rectangle, or diamond. These crystals can also form tube and oblong spherical type shapes. Crystals commonly identified by this lattice system are barite and olivine.

Monoclinic

This system uses three axes as well, but while the vertical axis meets the other two at a 90-degree angle, the two vertical axes meet each other at a corner that can be either larger or smaller than 90 degrees. These types of crystals usually consist of six faces and form long prisms. This is a very common lattice system for crystals, and some of the best examples are azurite, malachite, and pyroxene.

Triclinical

In this system, none of the three axes meet each other at a 90-degree angle. Unlike the six other lattice types, there is no symmetry to these crystals, and there are no faces that will mirror each other. There is also no regulation to the number of faces these crystals will have, although they do tend to be tubular. Some examples of triclinical crystals are axinite and plagioclase.

Crystal Shapes

A big part of crystal identification is the shape. The crystal lattice determines the potential types of shapes which can be identified by the number of faces, faces that mirror each other, and the basic symmetry of the crystal.

Although most crystals don't form geometrically perfect shapes, and crystals of the same type will not be identical in shape and size, they will conform to the same basic shape type. There are eleven basic shape types in which crystals can be classified.

Monohedron

This shape is also a pedion, and it consists of an undetermined number of faces that are each geometrically unique. None of the faces are parallel or mirror each other in any way. This shape is the result of a triclinic lattice.

Parallelohedron

This shape is another result of a triclinical lattice and can also be referred to as a pinacoid. This shape has two faces that run parallel to one another and are geometrically the same shape. These two faces might be a reflection or inversion of each other, but they are not perfectly mirrored.

Dihedron

A dihedron contains two faces that geometrically match and can either be related to each other through reflection or rotation. If these two faces are a simple reflection or rotation on only one axis, the dihedron will form a roughly dome-shaped crystal. If the two faces run along more than one rotational axis, the dihedron will form a more sphere-shaped crystal. The dihedron shape is caused by a monoclinic lattice type.

Disphenoid

The disphenoid shape consists of two sets of faces that are geometrically the same in shape and size, but they do not run parallel with each other. These shapes share symmetry through rotation and are connected by one of their edges. An orthorhombic lattice can result in a rhombic disphenoid, while a tetragonal lattice can result in a tetragonal disphenoid.

Prism

A prism consists completely of sets of mirroring faces that are both geometrically identical and run parallel to each other. The two faces of each mirroring set are on opposite sides of the crystal, and all the sets are reflected around the same axis. Usually, one set will form the base, which can be almost any basic shape, such as a square, triangle, or hexagon, while the other sets will all be rectangular. These rectangular faces that meet the edges of the base face at 90-degree angles will form a tube-like shape for the crystal. Prisms are a result of a monoclinic lattice system.

Pyramid

The pyramid shape consists of a base face and a set of three, four, six, eight, or twelve faces that do not run parallel to each other but meet in a point instead. Usually, the crystal will have a base face that can have one of several shapes, such as a square or triangle, with triangular shapes along each edge that will meet each other at the apex of the crystal. The shape of the base face will determine the type of pyramid and the number of faces in the set, and it is determined by the lattice type. The hexagonal, tetragonal, and orthorhombic lattice types are capable of producing pyramid-shaped crystals.

Dipyramid

This shape basically consists of two pyramids connected base to base with an apex at both ends. The two pyramids share the same base in the middle of the crystal and are a reflection of each other. A dipyramid shape can have a hexagonal, tetragonal, or orthorhombic lattice type, and the shape of the shared base will determine the type of dipyramid shape of the crystal. Each of the faces of a dipyramid will be triangular in shape as well, and a dipyramid will have twice as many faces as a pyramid with the same base.

Trapezohedron

A trapezohedron looks similar to a dipyramid but has significant differences. Firstly, a trapezohedron does not have a shared base between the two apexes of the shape. Rather than triangular shapes, each face will have a trapezoidal (four sides that are not perpendicular) shape. The type of trapezohedron will be determined by the amount of faces on each side (i.e. a trigonal trapezoid will have six faces in total, with three at the top and three at the bottom). A tetragonal trapezohedron will have four faces on both sides for a total of eight faces, and a hexagonal trapezohedron will have six faces on both sides, resulting in 12 faces. This shape can have a tetragonal or hexagonal lattice.

Scalenohedron

Like a trapezohedron, the scalenohedron resembles two pyramids but will have no base shape in the middle of the crystal. Unlike the trapezohedron, however, each of the faces of the crystal will be in the shape of a scalene triangle, meaning two of the corners of the triangle are smaller than 90 degrees and the other is larger than 90 degrees. A scalenohedron will have either eight or twelve faces that are grouped in symmetrical pairs. This shape can be the result of a hexagonal or tetragonal lattice.

Rhombohedron

This shape consists of six diamond-shaped faces and looks like a cube that is turned to stand upright on one corner and has been flattened or elongated along its diagonal axis. This shape can have a rhombohedral or hexagonal lattice type. An important trademark is that opposing sides of the rhombohedron are geometrically the same in shape and size and run parallel to each other; they are not a reflection of each other along a vertical or horizontal axis.

Tetrahedron

The tetrahedron is a shape composed of four triangular shapes. The lattice of the crystal will determine the type of tetrahedron and the shape of the triangle. A tetrahedron with an isometric lattice will consist of four equilateral (all three sides are the same length and all three corners are 60 degrees) triangles that are identical. A tetragonal lattice system will result in four identical triangles that each have two sides of the same length, also known as an isosceles triangle. A crystal with an orthorhombic lattice will have two sets of matching isosceles triangles.

Crystal Colors

Color is a large part of identifying crystals. The color of a crystal is mainly determined by the types of minerals the crystal is grown from, although many outside influences during the forming of a crystal can have a huge influence. Each crystal type has a certain lattice, growth process, and mineral composition, and each will have a specific color associated with it. Quartz is a good example in this case; a pure quartz crystal will be completely colorless, but outside influences can alter this. Amethyst is a member of the quartz family but gains its purple color from trace elements of iron within the crystal. Rose quartz is pink due to traces of titanium or manganese, and smoky quartz is brown because specific color centers are activated when traces of aluminum within the crystal are exposed to natural radiation transmitted by specific types of stone. Some crystal types will change colors if repeatedly exposed to light, such as realgar, which can change from red to yellow. Some crystals will change colors when viewed in different types of light, and crystals such as opal will reflect different colors when looked at from different angles. Many crystals and gemstones are often treated with intense heat when being transformed into jewelry as high temperatures can deepen the color of certain types.

These changes due to outside elements can be more intense in some crystal types and cause significant differences as seen with the quartz example, but in other crystal types, these changes are quite small, such as with azurite, where the exact hue of blue can be affected.

Certain colors will always be associated with specific elements and minerals, such as copper that will result in blue or green stones, iron that is usually associated with red and brown, and cobalt and manganese which can cause a pink hue. Due to this, certain colors in crystals will be linked to specific healing properties and uses.

Opacity and Transparency

When discussing the appearance of crystals, terms such as opaque, translucent, and transparent are bound to pop up. These three terms have everything to do with how much light passes through a crystal or how much light it reflects back. If a crystal is transparent, it means that all light passes through the crystal and you can see right through it with perfect clarity, just like glass. An opaque crystal reflects back all light and isn't see-through whatsoever. The term translucent is used when a crystal lets some light pass through but not all. These crystals can be partially seen through and are usually blurry.

The translucency of a crystal is mostly determined by the elements it is formed from but, once again, outside influences can have an effect on this. In some cases, it is even possible for one crystal to have varying degrees of translucency. Agate is a good example, as one ring can be completely transparent while the next can be only slightly translucent, bordering on opaque. Some crystal types have very reflective surfaces, though they do not fall into a classification of their own. Crystals with reflective surfaces can still be transparent, translucent, or opaque, depending on how much can be seen through the crystal beyond the reflection.

Stripes and Rings

Many crystal types such as tiger's eye, agate, and malachite are most easily recognized by their various layers of stripes and rings, and the intensity in the variations between the layers can often influence the value of these stones. All crystals, no matter how big or small, are formed in layers which are usually not noticeable by the human eye. Severe changes in the environment, such as temperature changes, the sudden appearance of new minerals, or a change in pressure, can cause small changes in the properties of a crystal, resulting in the current layer being a little bit different from the previous layer. Some minerals, such as chalcedony, are more sensitive to these changes and will form clearly varying layers more easily than others, becoming beautifully layered agate. The most common differences between layers are a change in the exact hue or intensity of the crystal's natural color or a shift in the opacity in each layer. Radical changes such as a blue and red layer in the same stone are not a natural occurrence. Many of these striped or ringed crystals are cut and polished in a way that will show off these layers as much as possible.

Imperfections

Growing crystals is a very complicated and precise process, and it's only natural for a few mistakes to be made here and there. Imperfections can have a large influence on the appearance and structural integrity of a crystal and make them either more or less valuable. Certain impurities can even have an influence on the healing properties of a crystal. There are different types of imperfections, namely impurities, interstitial defects, vacancy defects, displacement, and twinning. Impurities occur when an unwanted or incorrect type of atom is present within a crystal. A good example is lapis lazuli; this crystal is mostly made out of lazurite, but clusters of calcite and pyrite cause white and gold speckles. In the case of lapis lazuli, these impurities are preferred and make the crystal more valuable.

Interstitial defects happen when there is an extra atom within the lattice of the crystal where it doesn't belong. In opaque crystals, this is simply noticed by a small part that is a bit harder than the rest. In transparent and translucent crystals, this defect is more easily noticeable. This defect can be seen as a small part of the crystal looking more dense and opaque than the rest of it. Depending on the frequency and placement of these extra atoms, it can create misty swirls or darker veins within the crystal. Impurities can also be a type of interstitial defect if a different type of atom is squeezed into a space where no atoms belong.

A vacancy defect is the complete opposite and happens when there is an atom missing in the lattice pattern. A large number of vacancies spread throughout the crystal can cause it to be softer and more fragile than usual, but this is very rare. In most cases, the vacancies are small, and the structure of the atoms surrounding the vacancy will assure that the crystal does not collapse in on itself.

Dislocation occurs when there is a sudden shift in the lattice pattern of a crystal. This usually means that there is a partial plain or row added or removed from the pattern, and the rest of the lattice then moves slightly to maintain the stability of the crystal. In some cases, this can cause faint bends and wobbles in normally flat and straight surfaces on the crystal. These are usually so small, however, that they can't be seen by the naked eye.

Twinning basically happens when crystals of the same type are clustered too closely together and grow into one crystal. These are individual crystals that share some points in their lattice. A good example is pyrite, which has a cube shape. In the case of twinned pyrite, you will be able to see each individual cube, but they will be intersecting. These squares can either simply share a face, in which case they will simply look like two cubes roughly glued together, or they can penetrate each other, causing corners and edges of one cube to disappear into or grow out of the faces of the other cubes.

Cutting and Polishing

Crystals aren't always sold in the same state they are found in; they often go through a cleaning, cutting, and polishing process. When crystals are found or mined, they are treated beforehand to enhance their appearance, especially if they are destined to become jewelry. There are many different methods to cut and polish gems, but almost all involve the use of other, harder gemstones and crystals. Special tools such as saw-blades, grinders, and sandpaper are reinforced or created using incredibly hard crystals like diamond to cut and polish crystals into different shapes. Certain shapes also have special meanings and powers when used for healing. There are certain types of cuts that are used on more precious gemstones to show off their best attributes.

However, in many cases, it is popular to leave gems and crystals in a more natural shape. In these cases, the crystals are cut along their existing faces to remove any unattractive and extra bits or to reduce them to a more manageable size. It also often happens that these crystals are only very lightly polished or skip this step completely to achieve a very natural and rugged look. These crystals are called rough crystals.

A popular method of shaping and polishing crystals is a process called tumbling. Tumbling involves turning larger stones in a rotating barrel full of other, smaller crystals and stones. The smaller stones will begin softening the edges and smoothing the surface of the bigger crystals over time. The stones in which the crystal is rolled are regularly replaced with smaller and finer stones to get an even smoother look and feel. This process brings forth crystals with very interesting and beautiful organic shapes and can last for days, weeks, or even months. The longer the process lasts, the smoother and more rounded the crystal will become.

Crystals can still be bought in their original form, especially in stores specializing in their sales. These ones look quite different from their polished counterparts and can have a very interesting appearance. Crystals that aren't cut or polished are called raw crystals.

Chapter 2: An Abundance Of Crystals

Crystals have been adored and exalted for the past couple of centuries now by men and women alike because of their great beauty and their amazing molecular structure. They have been linked with the image of abundance, luxury and extreme wealth. Well, this is not entirely surprising because crystals are one of the rare solids that have a very uniform arrangement of particles. The arrangement of their particles is so organized that the manner in which they are structured can be considered geometric. It is like there is a mathematical equation hidden in each and every crystalline formation. That is why crystals are one of the very formidable and almost indestructible solids. That is also why most crystals are really precious, beautiful and valuable — making them as perfect emblems for high end ball gowns and dresses, state of the art watches, ridiculously expensive jewelries and exquisitely made masterpieces such as tiaras for queens and princesses. Crystals have earned their place in the world of luxury because they are not just beautiful in the outside but they are in the inside too.

There is another feature of crystals that make them a great tool in healing people's sickness and other health problems. This property is called resonance. Because of their geometric internal structure, crystals are thought to resonate at a specific frequency. It is the application of this resonance or vibration in an articulate manner that can trigger the natural healing processes and mechanisms that are built in our body system. They also say that crystals have this amazing capability to emit energies that can help the systems in our body work well in harmony. But before we can indulge ourselves with the in depth procedures of crystal healing, let us first look into the second, third and fourth step towards our crystal healing success, which is knowing the different kinds of crystal used in crystal healing, what they mean and what they are for.

Let us start with **Amethyst**. It is the birthstone of the people born on the month of February but it is more than just the birthstone of the February babies. Amethyst is considered to be the most helpful crystal used in crystal healing because the benefits of using this are universally applicable. It is also a great crystal to use if you want to meditate because it helps in clearing the mind and making the achieving peace and tranquility.

Then, there is the crystal called **Ruby**. The Ruby is a variant of the corundum, a very hard mineral which is also known as aluminum oxide. The Ruby can help rejuvenating the energies in the heart area as well maintain homeostasis within the anatomies of the body.

Another common favorite crystal in crystal healing is the **Rose Quartz Crystal.** It is the kind of crystal that gives off a calming and Zen-like effect. It can be used to make the body serene, as well as extract the latent and suppressed feelings to stop them from hindering your growth as a person.

The **Carnelian** is a favorite of Egyptians and we can totally see why. This crystal is an orange stone that can be commonly found in beaches. It is popularly known for the warm, cozy feeling that it exudes, as well as its revitalizing effect.

The **Topaz** is a crystal that can be used perfectly to redirect the energy that is flowing around your body. This crystal accomplishes this effect because it has an elongated form and parallel striations, making it a perfect crystal used in clearing.

The **Iron Pyrite** or what is popularly known as the "Fool's Gold" is a yellow stone used in crystal healing in order to put the digestive system at ease, as well as make the body cleansed and robust.

The **Bloodstone** is the kind of crystal that will help in stimulating emotional and personal growth. It also helps in circulating the blood properly around our system and making our heart healthy. It is a form of green quartz with hints of red jasper which makes it a perfect epitome of energy and equilibrium.

Another Egyptian favorite is the **Turquoise.** This crystal can be used in strengthening the systems of the body. This stone is used for protection and support.

If you are the shy type, the **Aquamarine** is the stone for you. This healing crystal can help improve confidence and can help the words that you have trouble and difficulty in saying easily out of your system.

The **Lapiz Lazuli**, another crystal used by the Egyptians, can help in releasing negative feelings and emotions such as stress out of your body. It can also help sweep off your mind from disturbing and negative thoughts.

The **Clear Quartz** is quite a popular crystal. In fact, it is one of the holiest stones during the ancient civilizations. It can strengthen the mind and the body. The clear quartz also symbolizes the power of the white light, and so, it is used as well as protection from negative energy.

The **Opal** is the most popular out of the multicolored stones because it works with the harmonization of emotion and feelings. It is also believed to be able to also balance with different chakras because it can reflect different colors.

The **Tourmaline** is one of those black crystals that can be perfectly used as protective stones. It is a good energy shifter and can help in realigning the problems concerning the bones and the skeleton.

The crystals discussed in the previous paragraphs are just a few of the many crystals used in crystal healing. Basically, the crystals are grouped together according to color as well and each color has a different purpose. Each color also corresponds to the different chakras in the body that they are associated or affiliated with.

The concept of chakras, as well as its locations in the different part of the body will be discussed in the succeeding chapters so for the time being, we will just discuss what the different color groups of crystal mean in the next chapter.

Chapter 3: How Do I Use Crystals To Heal Myself?

Whenever you're anxious or stressed out, your body's natural defenses become compromised. This makes you prone to acquiring illnesses. Healing must therefore begin through lowering your levels of stress.

How to Use Stress-relieving Crystals on your Chakras

In order to perform this method, you will require three amethyst crystals, four quartz crystals, one rose quartz, and two black onyx.

Place one amethyst crystal on your forehead (brow chakra). Meanwhile, the two other amethyst crystals are to be held in the palms of both your hands. The purpose of this is to create grounding, stabilizing, and calming effects through the chakras in your palms while increasing the flow of energy by guiding it upwards toward your crown chakra (the top of your head). Afterwards, the energy will be guided to descend back towards the root chakra (the base of your spine, around the tailbone).

The black onyx crystals are meant to be placed on the soles of your feet. They will help draw out all the stress-inducing negative energies away from your body and release them.

The rose quartz, on the other hand, is to be placed on your abdomen. This serves to create harmony between the male and the female energies (the yin and the yang). Furthermore, the rose quartz yields a rejuvenating effect.

Lastly, the four clear quartz crystals are to be arranged so that one is above your head and one is on your abdomen (solar plexus chakra). Place it just slightly higher than the rose quartz. Then, one clear quartz crystal should be placed on the left side of your arm and one on the right side of your arm. Clear quartz gemstones help to detoxify your aura and cleanse your chakras. They also restore balance and clarity.

When you place the healing stones as such, you are creating the Stress Reliever Crystal Pattern. This pattern creates two distinct triangle energy zones. The top triangle starts at the quartz crystal above your head and runs down the amethyst on your left hand, and then it connects horizontally to the amethyst in your right hand. The triangle is then completed with the line ascending towards the quartz on top of your head.

Meanwhile, the inferior triangle is made up of the healing stones placed on your abdomen which then descends to the crystal placed on your left foot. The line crosses towards the crystal on your right foot, and finally ascends to the rose quartz situated on your abdominal chakra.

To activate the power of these crystals, close your eyes and perform deep breathing. Observe as the air moves in and out of your body. Relax. Hold this state of relaxation for 10 minutes or when you're ready to come out of your tranquil state.

Afterwards, you may choose to carry these healing crystals wherever you go so that you may also use them as "worry stones". Place the healing stones in a pouch and keep them in your purse or in your pocket. Whenever you feel symptoms of stress or anxiety, take out the stones and rub them with your fingers.

What are the other ways to use healing crystals?

If the Stress Reliever Crystal Pattern isn't for you, don't worry. There are many other ways in which you can harness the stress-relieving energy of healing crystals. Read on and you're likely to find one that suits your preference as well as your daily routine.

Wear the healing crystals on your body or close to your body.

One of the ways in which you can utilize the healing energy of crystals is to wear them as jewelry. You can wear them as pendants or brooches or you may have them set on your ring. You may also keep them in small pouches pinned inside your clothes. This way, they can serve both as a tool for healing and as an amulet for protection. Crystal healing jewelry affects your energy field. It usually doesn't matter on which part of the body you wear the crystal but for a more concentrated effect, try carrying it as close as possible to the area which requires treatment. You may guide the crystal's healing energy by intention but some wearers choose to trust that the healing power will naturally flow towards where it is most needed.

When using the healing crystal as a pendant, the length of the chain is something that you should consider well. For instance, a short chain will allow the crystal to rest on your throat chakra. Therefore, the stone's effect will be more concentrated on areas governed by that particular chakra such as communication and the treatment of illnesses around the neck area. Meanwhile, a longer chain will allow the healing crystal pendant to come in contact with your chest. Thus, the stone will have a more powerful effect on areas covered by the heart chakra such as compassion and love. Nevertheless, the stone will still be able to supply energy to your entire aura and to the rest of your body.

Furthermore, there are those who feel that when healing crystals are worn on the left side of the body, they tend to concentrate more on receiving energy. Meanwhile, wearing the stones on the right side of the body appears to be more helpful in external issues.

Keep the healing crystals under your pillow.

Having healing stones beneath the pillow will aid individuals who are suffering from insomnia and other sleep pattern disturbances. They are also effective in warding off bad dreams. Some healing crystals like the garnet possess properties that can assist you in dream recall. There are also those that can aid you in astral travel.

Use healing crystals in the bath.

Healing crystals can also be added to your bathwater. Alternatively, you may arrange them around the edges of the tub. This provides you with a pleasant and calming environment while you bathe. This is important because bathing does not only serve to cleanse the physical form. Bathing cleanses you on various levels. The act helps in washing away the stresses that have accumulated during the day as well as all the undesirable emotions that you have been harboring within you. When you place crystals in or on the bath, it will absorb all these negative energies. Thus, this ensures that your bath will have a complete soothing, revitalizing, and energizing effect. The most ideal crystals to incorporate in your bath include aventurine, rose quartz, and clear quartz.

Use healing crystals while meditating.

The healing crystal's energy structure organically provides stillness and harmony. This is why it's effective in calming the mind. What most people fail to realize is that problems are merely matters that have not been fixed by one's regular thought processes. By modifying your manner of thinking, one can easily find solutions to these problems. If you are in the habit of meditating, healing crystals may be used by holding them in the palm of your hands or by setting them in front of you.

Arrange healing crystals around your home or your workspace.

This will effectively cleanse the room and clear the space since crystals have the capacity to change the energy of an environment. They are useful in energizing the general aura of any room as well as in neutralizing negative energies. Furthermore, gemstones inspire harmony. When arranging the healing stones in your room, be sure to follow your intuition. It might be important to note that raw crystals are known to be more capable of retaining the integrity of their own energy. Hence, they are more effective in absorbing and trapping in negative energies. This means that they require less frequent cleansing compared to smaller single gemstones.

Chapter 4: Beginning Of Crystal Healing

It's reasonable to say that as long as we've been a species, we've had an affinity with rocks and crystals. The use of talismans and amulets goes back to the origins of the human race, although we have no manner of understanding how the first of these artifacts were regarded or used. Many early parts were of organic origin. Beads sculpted from mammoth ivory were collected from a tomb in Sungir, Russia, 60,000 years ago (Upper Palaeolithic era), as well as modern beads produced from the shell and fossil shark teeth.

Crystal Healing has a lengthy, colorful past. Doctors, shamans, magicians, priests and healers utilized the energy of crystals in many ways.

Tribal societies handled rocks in ingenious ways, to predict the future, to interact with the ancestors and to cure illnesses.

Antique Egyptian civilizations used prolific healing crystals. Native American cultures have created comprehensive use of the protection and healing energy of many crystals. These and numerous other countries were in contact with the soil, the environment and their position as human beings in the natural world. Over the last five thousand years, mystics and magic have repeatedly told us that we belong to the world as mountains and trees. We disregard their wisdom in our peril.

The oldest amulets are Baltic amber, discovered 20,000 years ago. Amber beads were also discovered in Britain 10,000 years ago. The distance they traveled to Britain demonstrates the individuals of that moment their worth. Jet was also common and jet earrings, bracelets and necklaces were found in Palaeolithic tombs in Belgium and Switzerland. Malachite mines were proven to exist in Sinai as early as 4000 BC.

Amulets were prohibited by the Christian clerks in 355 AD, but gemstones continued to serve a significant part, with Saphir being the favorite gem for ecclesiastical seals in the 12th century. Marbodus, Bishop of Rennes in the 11th century, asserted that agate would make the wearer more pleasing, persuasive and for God's sake.

Historical References

The first historical references to the exploitation of crystals originate from the old Sumerians, who created magic formulas incorporating them. Ancient Egyptians used lapis lazuli, turquoise, carnelian, coral and transparent quartz in their jewelry. They sculpted tomb amulets of the same gems, too. Egyptians used rocks mainly to protect and preserve their health. Chrysolite (subsequently known as Topaz or Peridot) was known to help fighting night terror and drowning evil spirits. Egyptians made use of crystals in cosmetology as well. Galena (which is a lead metal) was crushed and was used as an eye shadow later labeled as "kohl". Another stone that has been used in a similar manner is malachite. Green rocks, in particular, were used to indicate the core of the dead and were included in the tombs. Green rocks were used contemporary in Ancient Mexico.

Ancient Greeks ascribed many characteristics to gemstones and lots of the denominations we now use have Greek origins. The term 'crystal' originates from the Greek 'ice' because it was thought that transparent quartz was water that had cooled so deeply, that it would always stay strong. The term amethyst implies 'not drunk' and was carried as remedy for intoxication and hangovers. Hematite was named after 'blood' because of the coloring it produces when it oxidizes. Hematite is iron ore and the ancient Greeks linked iron with the god of battle, Aries. Greek fighters would rub hematite all over their bodies, apparently to render themselves indestructible. Greek seamen also carry a range of amulets to protect them at sea.

Jade was extremely prized in ancient China and some Chinese characters represented jade crystals. Musical instruments in the shape of chimes were produced of jade and some 1000 years ago Chinese emperors were sometimes placed in jade armor. There are jade mask weddings in Mexico around the same period. Jade has been recognized as a healing rock for the kidneys in both China and South America. Around 250 years ago the indigenous population of New Zealand, known as Māori, wore jade pendants depicting ancestor spirits, which were handed down through the masculine line for many centuries. The tradition of fortunate green rocks remains to this day in areas of New Zealand.

Crystals in Religion

Crystals and gemstones were used in a way or another in all religions. They are referenced throughout the Bible, in the Koran and many other spiritual documents. The source of the birthstones is the breastplate of Aaron, or the "High Priest Breastplate," as stated in the Book of Exodus. The 4th of the seven Heavens in the Koran consists of a carbuncle (garnet). The Kalpa Tree, which constitutes an invitation to the gods in Hinduism, is said to have been built completely of precious stone and the Buddhist text of the 7th century mentions a diamond altar located close the Tree of Knowledge (the neem tree under which Siddhartha meditated). A thousand Kalpa Buddhas rested on this seat. The Kalpa Sutra, in Jainism, talks of Harinegamesi, the holy captain of the foot soldiers who captured 14 precious stones, cleansed them of their lower characteristics and kept only their best nature to help their changes.

There is also an old sacred lapidary text, the Ratnapariksha of Buddhatta. Some sources say it's Hindu, but it's most probable Buddhist. The period is unsure, but it's likely from the 6th century. Diamonds in this book are extremely regarded as the King of gemstones and are classified by caste. The Sanskrit term for diamond, vajra, is also the term for the Hindu goddess Indra and diamonds are often linked with thunder. The ruby was also greatly admired. It was an inextinguishable flame and it was intended to preserve the physical and mental health of the wearer. The treaty lists many other gemstones and their characteristics.

The Renaissance

In Europe, from the 11th century to the Renaissance, a variety of medical treatises extolled the merits of precious and semi-precious stones in the therapy of certain diseases. Typically, rocks have been used along with herbal antidotes. The creators were Hildegard von Binghen, Arnoldus

Saxo and John Mandeville. References are also made to stones with specific power or safety characteristics. In 1232 Hubert de Burgh, prime justice of Henry III, was convicted of taking a gem from the king's treasury, which would render the wearer powerless and give it to Llewellyn, the King of Wales and Henry's foe. It was also thought that the gemstones were damaged by Adam's initial sins, that they might be populated by demons, or that if they were to be treated by a sinner, their qualities would disappear. Therefore, before carrying, they should be sanctified and consecrated. Today, there are reminiscences of this faith in the purification and programming of crystals before use in crystal healing.

The tradition of using precious stones in healing was still recognized during the Renaissance, but the inquiring minds of the era attempted to figure out how the method truly functioned and to offer it a more academic explanation.

The Beginning of Crystal Healing

In 1609 Anselmus de Boot, a court doctor of Rudolf II of Germany stateed that any virtue of a gemstone should be due to the existence of nice or bad angels. The good angels would bestow unique grace upon the gems, but the evil angels would tempt individuals to believe in the rock itself and not in the donations of God conferred upon it. He continues to mention some rocks as useful and to lay down the characteristics of others merely to superstition. Later in the same century, Thomas Nicols expressed in his 'Faithful Lapidary' that crystals, as lifeless objects, could not have had the impact believed in the past. Thus, in the Age of Enlightenment, the use of precious stones for healing and security started to drop out of favor in Europe.

A variety of exciting studies were performed in the beginning portion of the 19th century to show the impacts of rocks on people who thought themselves to be clairvoyant. In one instance, the topic asserted not only to feel physical and mental modifications when touched by multiple rocks but also to experience scents and flavors.

Crystal and Gemstone Meaning

In spite of no longer being in medicinal use, gemstones have persisted in having significance. Until lately, the jet was popularly carried by those in mourning and the grenade was often carried in wartime. There is a tradition in the local community here in the north of England: every woman descendant carries an antique moonstone necklace for her wedding, which has been in the community for centuries. It was only later that one family member realized that it was a sign of fertility.

Many indigenous societies have persisted in using gemstones for healing up till recent times, if not until today. The Zuni tribe in New Mexico is making fetishes of rock, representing animal spirits. They were ceremonially' fed' on powdered turquoise and ground maize. Beautiful inlaid fetishes are still produced for sale and are very collectible artifacts or carvings, although the spiritual practice that surrounds them is no longer very much in use. Other native American groups still retain sacred precious stones, particularly turquoise. Both Aborigines and Maoris have traditions concerning rocks and medicine or spiritual practice, some of which they share with the remainder of the globe, while some information remains personal within their societies.

It is essential not to forget that there are many instances of gemstones meaning comparable stuff to distinct societies, even though there has been no contact between these societies and no chance for a crossover. Jade was considered a remedy for kidney disorders by ancient Chinese, as well as by the Aztec and Mayan civilizations. Turquoise used to be worn to attract strength and health and jaspers have almost always delivered stability and calmness.

A New Age Dawns

In the 1980s, with the emergence of New Age culture, the utilization of crystals and precious stones started to re-emerge as a technique of healing. Much of the practice has been taken from ancient traditions, with more data coming from testing and channeling. Katrina Rafael's books in the '80s and Melody and Michael Gienger's books in the '90s revived the use of stones.

Nowadays, a big amount of novels are accessible on the topic and crystals are frequently featured in magazines and newspaper articles. Crystal therapy crosses the limits of Christian and spiritual belief. Not perceived as a domain of alternative culture anymore, it is now seen as an appropriate and more popular complementary treatment and many schools are now offering it as a qualifying topic.

Chapter 5: How Crystal Healing Works

There is a wide range of hypotheses encompassing whether crystal healing works and how they work. Indeed, even the historical backdrop of crystal healing has an assortment of convictions, running from old Egyptian practices to cutting edge Chinese and Buddhist practice

The most well-known hypothesis is that it originates from the Chinese idea of chi, which is life-energy, and Buddhist convictions encompassing chakras. These chakras are accepted to associate the spiritual components to the physical elements of the body.

The fundamental chakra focuses are as per the following:

The forehead

Over the head

Throat

Stomach

Chest

Genitals

The situation of specific crystals on the chakra focuses related to whatever sickness or stress you have is said to realign the life-energy and help to heal by offsetting the energy. Notwithstanding, you can likewise wear individual crystals to support you or place them underneath your pad around evening time to pick up similar advantages.

In the same way as other different types of elective medication, how powerful crystals may assist you with healing will rely upon your very own convictions and confidence. If you think something will work, it is bound to do as such. If you have negative musings encompassing the use of crystals, for example, non-accepting their forces, they are more reluctant to work.

Another significant thing to recall is that there is a lot of varying feelings out there concerning what every crystal speaks to. Additionally, a crystal may not work the equivalent for one individual than another. Fortunately, there are frequently determinations of crystals that work on similar zones, so it might be a little experimentation to locate the correct one that suits and works for you.

Chapter 6: The World Of Crystals

What is Crystal?

A crystal is a material formed by solidification of chemicals and has a regularly repeating internal arrangement of atoms and molecules. This highly ordered structure forms a crystal lattice extending in all directions. The crystal lattice, which is balanced and orderly, emits a consistent energy. When a crystal comes into contact with a dissonant energy, the crystal transforms that chaotic energy into a harmonic energy. The ability to "bring order to chaos" forms the basis for the healing and spiritual power of crystal.

Geometrical Shapes

Crystals come in a variety of geometrical shapes – a result of internal compression. Crystals come in all shapes, from tumbled stones and cut crystals to natural formations like clusters, wands and phantoms. For example:

Mineralogical samples are crystals still on their rock base, i.e. in the form in which they were found;

Crystal clusters are a number of crystals sharing a common base;

Single crystals are recognized by their geometric shapes; and

Tumbled stones are damaged crystals polished by gravels.

Tumbled Stones

Metaphysical Function

A crystal's shape may determine its metaphysical function. For example:

Abundance crystals are large crystals with an abundance of small crystals clustered around their base. This type of crystal can be used when you want to multiply something, e.g. money.

Clusters are group of crystals that have grown together on the same base. This kind of crystal symbolizes community. Clusters can be used when you are dealing with issues concerning cooperation, harmony, union and friendship.

Channeling crystals are clear, quartz crystals typically having at least one, large, seven-sided face on one side of their tip, and a triangular three-sided face on the other. These make good tools for meditation, allowing those using them to stay open to insights and inspirations that come "out of the blue".

Color

Crystals are perhaps best known for their color, which is determined by the internal arrangement of atoms. Although many minerals are colorless in their pure state, impurities of the atomic structure give crystals their color. Understanding the symbolism of color is of paramount importance. For example:

Red is the color of passion and blood. It stands for anger or alarm. Use red crystals if you feel especially passionate about an issue or if you need to boost your courage, sexual attraction or passion.

Red crystal examples: Alexandrite, fire opal, garnet, red carnelian, red jasper, red tourmaline, rhodochrosite, ruby.

Orange is a warm, cheerful color, offering optimism and hope. Use orange crystals when you want to stimulate mental power, optimism or feelings of abundance.

Orange crystal examples: Amber, orange calcite, orange carnelian, sunstone, tiger's eye, topaz.

Yellow is radiant and bright like the sun. Yellow crystals relate to intelligence. When in their vicinity, your mind works better and you find it easier to focus. Yellow crystals can be used when wishing to express joy and happiness or lift melancholy.

Yellow crystal examples: Ametrine, citrine, golden calcite, goldstone, pyrite, sunstone, tiger's eye, topaz, yellow jasper.

Blue, the color of the sky inspires tranquility and is good for meditation and intuition. Use blue crystals if trying to connect to your subconscious or if searching for inspiration.

Blue crystal examples: Angelite, azurite, blue lace agate, blue obsidian, labradorite, lapis lazuli, sapphire, tanzanite.

Green is the color of Nature and symbolizes harmony and peaceful, healthy existence. Use green crystals to stimulate inner peace and healing.

Green crystal examples: Aventurine, emerald, green calcite, green fluorite, green obsidian, green tourmaline, jade, malachite, moldavite.

Black can represent seriousness, darkness, depression, death, etc. You can use black crystals when fighting addictions, or when dealing with hidden, occult or mysterious issues.

Black crystal examples: Apache tears, black pearls, black tourmaline, Boji stones, obsidian, and onyx.

Shapes

It's necessary to understand the importance of the shapes in which crystals come. While some are natural, many are shaped in workshops to can serve a certain purpose. For certain practices, the type of crystal is very important as it further enhances the results you want to achieve.). For example:

Healing massage wands are smooth, palm-size pieces that fit nicely in the hand. They are rounded at one end to run smoothly over the body, and pointed at another to be used for acupressure and chakra healing. They are used to channel energy in reflexology and massage. The stone should be chosen for its particular benefits and energies.

Chakra Healing

Obelisks are four-sided pillars that terminate in a pyramid shape. Symbolically, an obelisk can discharge tension through its tip and send it high into atmosphere to be dissipated. It can also draw energy from the upper atmosphere and ground that energy through its base.

Pyramids can be used to focus and to ground energy. They also have the power to absorb negative energy and blockage from the chakras. A gemstone pyramid is also used to enhance and to focus the inherent properties of the stone of which it is made.

Spheres and crystal balls symbolize the cyclical nature of life. Circles symbolize infinity because they have no beginning and no end. Spheres/balls are usually used for healing and rituals.

Tumbled stones have no rough edges and are convenient for laying on in healing sessions or grid work. Besides, they are convenient to carry.

Crystal clusters bring harmony. Clusters such as Quartz crystals clusters have been used for healing, meditation and expanding the mind to touch the spirit world.

Most of the crystals used today are minerals created about 5 billion years ago when the Earth was being formed. The rocks where these crystals are found are mixtures of different minerals and are classified as:

Igneous: formed when lava cooled and solidified (e.g. lava rocks in Hawaii);

Sedimentary: formed through accumulation of sediments of other rocks, usually in seas and oceans (e.g. Grand Canyon in Arizona); or

Metamorphic: formed when rocks were forced to change their shape and composition due to exposure to tremendous heat or pressure (e.g. the Scottish Highlands).

What Does All this Mean?

Crystals are formed deep within the earth, forced to grow under intense pressure and are structured according to precise mathematical rules, adhering to clearly-defined geometric patterns. Yet, they are all unique, each one carrying individual energy and qualities. They can be used for technology, divination, and self-development and healing. If you look after them and learn how to program them, they can help you find answers to all the questions you might ever face.

As Isabel Walbourne so beautifully put it, "May crystals give you power."

Crystals, Minerals, Rocks and Gemstones

Terms like crystals, minerals, rocks and gemstones are often used interchangeably, however, each of these solids exhibits significant characteristics distinguishing it from the others. The differences are not always easy to spot or to explain.

Minerals are naturally occurring, solid chemical compounds formed slowly as part of the geological process. Each mineral has a specific chemical composition, and is made of one or more elements. Minerals can be pure elements or complex chemical compounds.

Simply put, rocks are made of minerals. When you look at a rock and see different colors, you are seeing the minerals of which the rock is composed. To date, over 3,000 minerals have been identified.

Some of the most common minerals are quartz, gypsum, Sulphur, and fluorite.

Crystals, on the other hand, are structures comprised of ions, atoms and molecules all arranged in a repeating pattern. This process is called crystallization. Crystals start off as liquid particles that eventually solidify. The structure of the crystal depends on the chemistry of the fluid from which it is formed. Crystals can only be formed when atoms, molecules or ions are packed under pressure.

So, minerals are naturally occurring materials while crystals are comprised of a variety of different natural materials.

Some of the best known crystals are: amethyst, bloodstone, carnelian, citrine, lapis lazuli, and moonstone.

Rocks are not minerals. They can be an aggregate of one or more minerals, or not composed of minerals at all. There are three main rock types: igneous (basalt, granite), sedimentary (chalk, limestone, shale) and metamorphic (marble, quartzite, slate).

Gemstones (also called precious stones, jewels, gems) are pieces of mineral crystal that, when cut and polished, are used to make jewelry. They can be divided into precious (diamond, ruby, sapphire and emerald) and semi-precious stones (all other gemstones, such as opal, topaz, carnelian, rose quartz, turquoise, lapis lazuli, and many others). They are characterized with distinctive color or clarity.

Uses of Crystal

Crystals are well-known for their technological, healing and metaphysical qualities. Scientists and spiritual believers both claim to know how crystals work and their opinions usually clash.

Crystals in Technology

One of the most fascinating characteristics of certain crystals is that they produce an electrical charge when compressed. This is known as the piezoelectric effect and was discovered in the 19th Century by Pierre and Jacques Curie. Eventually, with the development of science, it was possible to put this discovery to use, e.g. in record player needles and a variety of measuring devices. Today, such devices "are used in almost every conceivable application requiring accurate measurement and recording of dynamic changes in mechanical variables such as pressure, force and acceleration."

Crystals transmit a piezoelectric charge that affects the body's bio-magnetic fields. Crystals reflect and retract light/light rays such as infrared and ultraviolet rays, which are both used to heal and to disinfect the body. Crystals also have the power to carry information. **(Why do you think every computer in the world contains a silicon (crystal) chip?)** Even from a scientific standpoint, it seems possible natural crystals can influence physical functioning.

It would be hard to imagine life without crystals since they play a very important role in electronics and optical industries. It is safe to say technological development without crystals would not be possible. Here are some examples of the ways modern science uses crystals:

Solar Cells (powering instruments from calculators to space vehicles);

Transistors (based on the same types of materials and crystals as solar cells, transistors can regulate electron flow, and amplify radio signals and act as digital switches);

Liquid Crystals (wrist watches, some type of clocks and pocket calculators use liquid crystals);

Protein Structures (crystals help solve different protein structure, which is very useful in biochemistry);

Pencils (graphite is a type of crystal);

Computer Chips (silicones form the basis for all microelectronics, such as computer chips);

Optical Equipment (some optical equipment is made from crystals);

CD's and DVD's (crystalline solids in CD's and DVD's enable us to write and to store information on them).

Crystals in Metaphysics

Metaphysics is hard to define since, broadly speaking, it refers to "everything that is unseen." So, it can refer to healing, psychic development, angels, ghost hunting, meditation, mediumship, channeling, shamanism, etc.

Metaphysics deals with abstract concepts most of which defy measurement and can, therefore, not be scientifically proven. Although ancient cultures considered metaphysics a science, in this day and age, it can best be described as a philosophy, at least until its concepts become testable.

On the other hand, many believe metaphysics is at the forefront of physics because it explores new, unchartered territories of thought until science has the tools to examine and test them. Only then can metaphysical teachings gain scientific approval. Until such a time, metaphysics will continue to explore the mysteries of the Universe by thinking "out of the box" and by approaching all questions with an open mind.

The underlying theme of the New Age Movement is spiritual development and, therefore, popular metaphysical topics resonate strongly with the New Age outlook on spirituality, consciousness and health.

Topics explored by metaphysics include:

Psychic Development

Spiritual Growth

Meditation

Working with Angels and Spirit Guides

Astral and Out-of Body Travelling

Divination Systems such as Tarot, Astrology and Numerology

The Power of Crystals

Feng Shui

Past Life Regression

Alternative Healing

The Law of Attraction

Crystals play a significant role in most of these disciplines. In ancient civilizations, as well as in the New Age movement today, crystals were believed to possess spiritual properties representing different energies that could be harnessed through their use. Although science remains skeptical, studies have shown crystals do have some sort of effect on the human body.

The bottom line is, all these techniques require raised consciousness, an open mind and positive energy. In the text below I've listed some of the crystals believed effective in certain areas:

Psychic Abilities

Consistent use of crystals can help develop and enhance these abilities. Crystals possess powerful energies, which can help correct unbalanced vibrations in the body. The most common crystals used by psychics, as well as those who want to achieve higher consciousness and establish communication with spiritual realm, are:

Amethyst - enhances psychic abilities and is also good as a psychic protection tool. It vibrates to the frequencies of the third eye and the crown chakras, and is often used in preparation for psychic readings.

Turquoise is an excellent enhancer of clairvoyant abilities. It's been suggested that stronger psychic powers will emerge when carrying and working with turquoise. It can be used to cleanse the body's energy centers and balance and open all the chakras. Turquoise helps spiritual attunement, is good for psychic protection and for keeping negative energies at a distance.

Bloodstone heightens psychic abilities and intuition. Many psychics consider this powerful stone magical. It's believed to give protection from evil. It's also used to release blockages in the subtle body.

Meditation

Meditation is beneficial to every aspect of your being: physical, mental, emotional and spiritual. It helps relax the body, slowing heart rate and lowering blood pressure. It relieves stress and quiets the mind. Through meditation, we release negative emotions and achieve a greater sense of awareness.

You'll be surprised how much you can understand about life when you sit in silence. For some reason, silence gives you a distance and you suddenly start seeing things, and people, in new and clearer ways.

Crystals most often used to assist meditation are blue stones such as aquamarine, blue calcite and turquoise as they have a calming effect on human mind. You can also use purple and clear stones, such as amethyst and clear quartz to help you reach higher states of consciousness.

In order to absorb the calming properties of a crystal during meditation, you can hold small crystals in your hands or wear crystal jewelry during meditation. Alternatively, you can place a crystal in front of you and use it as something on which to focus your attention. Some people place stones on the heart chakra (for emotional balance) or on the third eye chakra (for mental clarity) during meditation.

Feng Shui

Crystals are very popular with feng shui practitioners by helping to create good energy in the area where they are placed.

Specific crystals are used for specific energy, e.g. calming, energizing or to help one concentrate. When placed correctly, crystals help clear negative energy, thus enabling positive energy to take over, which in turn raises your vibrations and attracts good things in life.

To gain the maximum protection and help from crystals, consult feng shui books or consultants. You will learn to identify the location of the five elemental components in your living space around which feng shui practice revolves a – fire, water, earth, metal and wood.

Once you identify key areas of your environment, you can place the right crystals to allow positive energies in and to reduce or dispel bad energies. Positive energy in your living or working environment helps bring success and dissipate bad luck.

Many crystals can help improve the energy of your living space, but if ever in doubt, or if you can't afford to buy crystals of different types and colors, it's safe to use clear quartz.

Past Life Regression

Past life regression is a method of hypnosis allowing one to tap into past lives.

As these are very personal and private activities, it is probably best to use crystals that will relax, calm and help you focus, e.g. blue apatite, indigo quartz, amethyst, clear quartz, etc.

The Law of Attraction

There are crystals and stones to help you achieve your dreams. The trick is to choose the right ones for each specific goal. Keep your selected stones on or near you all the time (especially during visualization) or keep them somewhere where you can easily, and often, see them. Here are a few suggestions:

To get a new job, try using citrine (associated with wealth and prosperity), amazonite (improves self-worth and increases confidence), and agate (helps keep you strong and courageous) or peridot brings vitalizing energy. The most important thing is to stay positive.

Boosting creativity can come from smoky quartz, rainbow obsidian, and carnelian.

Improved health can be achieved with the help of turquoise, tourmaline or clear quartz.

To heal relationships, use white calcite.

Finding new love is helped by rose quartz.

Increase positive thinking by using amethyst, watermelon tourmaline or agate.

Medicinal Crystals

Healers, shamans and priests have long used crystals for their unique and special properties.

Although we are not certain how crystals work, we know that energy fields of crystals are influenced by their geometrical form, color and subtle vibrations. When choosing crystals for healing purposes, it's very important to pay attention to their form, shape and color.

Unlike us, ancient traditions were very observant of everything going on around them, and noticed that the presence of certain crystals promoted different kinds of medical benefits. For example:

Amethyst possessed calming effect and was effective to treat headaches;

Aquamarine helped regulate the immune system and heart; known as a stone of courage, in ancient times it was used to ward off dark energy and bring protection.

Carnelian helped boost energy and the reproductive system;

Citrine was good for purification on all levels, and particularly with cleansing the spleen, kidneys and liver; it also helped lift one's energy and spirits;

Emeralds help with the problems related to thymus and childbirth;

Jade helped with cleansing the blood and the nervous system;

Rubies assisted with cholesterol and blood clots problems;

Sapphire helped in case of inflammation and fever.

Choosing a Crystal that's Right for You

How to Choose a Crystal?

When buying crystals, you may want to buy a specific type, color or shape for the purpose you need. Sometimes, however, you are inexplicably drawn to certain crystals which "catch your eye" and you buy them even if you don't know what they are. If you hold such a crystal in your hand, you may even feel a greater urge to own it.

When this happens, it means you and the crystal are on the same "wave length". The crystal "called to you" because it probably also wanted to belong to someone with a matching energy.

There are hundreds of books on the subject regarding which crystal is good for what, but I think you can achieve much better results if you work with a crystal you can match to your energy. Crystals are living beings and we should treat them as such. Who would you rather have as a roommate - Someone good looking, bright and well-known or someone with whom you have a lot in common?

We know that everything around us vibrates at a particular frequency. So when choosing a crystal choose the one whose vibration matches your own. However, vibrations are not constant, they change all the time, which explains why at some stage of your life you may find pink crystal attractive, while at another you only go for yellow ones.

Crystals which match our own vibration frequency can be used to raise our vibrations and make us feel good.

On the other hand, if you have a crystal near you and it is not a good match, it will constantly drain you by lowering your vibration frequency. Therefore, selecting the right crystal is very important, especially if you are going to keep it near you or wear it as jewelry.

Cleaning your Crystal

Once you bring a new crystal home, the first thing you need to do is clean it. That's necessary as you want to remove the energy of all those who held it in the shop, many of whom may have inadvertently passed on their negative energy. Besides, the crystal may have travelled thousands of miles before it got to the shop.

This particularly applies to quartz crystals since they easily attract all kinds of "vibrations". Crystals, being living organisms, are "open" to receiving all kinds of energies from their environment. So, before starting to use the stone, and even before displaying it in your home or office, first remove any unwanted energies, which might have accumulated from the moment it was dug out from the earth. Cleaning is particularly important if stones you buy are second-hand and were used by someone else.

Advice for cleaning crystals range from washing it with plain water, with soap or mild detergent, keeping it in salty water, exposing it to the mid-day sun (for disinfection and energy absorption) or moonlight (for drawing in spiritual energy), keeping it buried in ground for a couple of days (so the Earth extracts the negative energy), etc. All I can say is that I managed to destroy many beautiful crystals by following this advice.

The best way to clean a crystal is to keep it under running tap water for a couple of minutes and hope all the negative energy it may have accumulated, be dispelled. You shouldclean all your crystals at least once a month, and if you use them for healing others, I suggest you clean them after each session, so as not to pass on whatever energy may have accumulated.

But, whatever you decide to do, DO NOT keep crystals in a water/ salt mixture or expose them to the mid-day sun!

Tune In to your Crystal

Here are 3 simple steps to find out if a crystal works for you:

Relax, remove all distractors (and pets) from the room and breathe slowly;

Hold a crystal in your hand, see how it feels against your skin; give yourself couple of minutes;

State your intention (to get a job, to be healthy, to find love, etc.). If the crystal is "responding" you will know it – you will catch yourself smiling, feeling light or just happy without any reason. If such cases, you've found a loyal friend!

If nothing happens, don't worry. It could mean you chose the wrong crystal, or you still have to learn the art of tuning-in. Practice meditation for a few days, then try again. Or, try with a different stone. In any case, don't give up.

Chapter 7: Choosing Your Crystals

All crystals and crystal stones should be rinsed before using them. You have no clue where they have been, who has been getting them to check whether they were a privilege fit for their energy fields or what kinds of energies are as of now joined to them. So the first thing you have to do when you get them home is to wash down them!

There are a couple of different approaches to cleanse your new crystals. You can use smirching, water cleansing, Mother Earth's energy, sage tea healing, sunlight based energy, sound vibrations, reflect the energy, and even sand healing if you pick.

To wash down your crystals with smearing, hold the crystal inside the smoke of your smirch stick. Smirching with pure savvy or a bright mix works best for crystal healing. Pass them through the smear smoke, at any rate, multiple times to and fro.

Cleansing your crystal with water and ocean salt is straightforward. For the harder crystals, you can put them in a little glass compartment of ocean saltwater for at any rate 60 minutes. For the smoother crystals, you can mist them liberally with a water shower to totally cover the crystal and having a lot of run-offs.

Using Mother Earth's energy is a straightforward and fun; yet filthy way to rinse your crystals. Take your crystal and enclose it by a straightforward cheesecloth and afterward again in a material made of silk. Locate a beautiful place in your yard where you can cover your new crystal. Burrow an opening around 6-8 creeps into the ground and place your crystal in this. Spread it and make sure to put a marker so you can uncover it! Following a time of 24 hours, reveal your crystal and delicately flush any free earth from it.

Sage tea cleansing is a safe and fun approach to fuse a couple of various angles together for a fantastic healing session for your crystals. Take some savvy, crisp if you have it, and mix a pot of tea produced using the new wise. Enable this to cool and place your crystal in a glass bowl. Pour the sage implanted tea over the crystal and enable it to wash medium-term. This joins the quality of smearing and water energy to cleanse them. Make sure to wash them in the first part of the day!

Sun based energy and water can also be used for cleansing crystals. You can achieve this by holding the crystal under running water for a moment and afterward putting the crystal in the sun to dry. A few crystals may blur with the immediate beams of the sun, so try not to leave them in the immediate daylight for a really long time. It just takes a couple of moments for them to dry, so watch out for them!

Healing Your Crystals

The use of sound vibrations is another superb method to rinse crystals with pure sound. A chime or tuning fork can be used for this. Use your chime or tuning fork to make its vibrational sound and place the crystal as close as you can to the ringer or tuning fork without intruding on the sound vibrational.

Using mirror energy to scrub crystals and crystal stones is extremely simple. Just place your crystal over a mirror, set on your table or dresser, and enable the mirror to reflect back and out the energy that the crystal is as of now holding. Enable this to stay on the mirror for at any rate 24 hours.

You can likewise use a sand technique for practically any sort of crystal or crystal stone. Cover your crystal in wet sand and leave for in any event 2 hours. Kindly note that the sand can expel a portion of the clean from the crystals, so just use this if all else fails.

When working with crystals in healing sessions, or even with crystal gridding, you will need to ensure you cleanse them all the time. Each issue is unique and should be considered relying upon what the healing or gridding is achieving with its errand. One fundamental dependable guideline, ensure you heal your crystals after every individual healing session. When working with system gridding alignments, these can fluctuate from healing once per week to once a month's time spans. Crystals that are worn ought to be purified and afterward reconstructed at regular intervals if need be. If you don't mind, follow the rules in this book for the best outcomes.

If you use crystal healing chip away at a predictable premise, regardless of whether it is for yourself or different healings, recollect that the crystals are the ones doing the healing work. It is continuously a smart thought to send them home to Mother Earth for at any rate one month during a schedule year when they are used this frequently. By this, I intend to cover them in Mother Earth to give them their very own energizing vibrational healing. Make sure to stamp the place where you hid them and write in your schedule to remind you when to reveal them once more!

Chapter 8: Choosing The Right Crystal

Being a newbie in the realm of crystal healing, one of the first lessons to learn is how to choose the right crystal for yourself and/or for the chosen purpose. The trick is this statement, 'You don't choose crystals. They choose you!'

Finding the Right Crystals in a Brick-and-Mortar Store Using Your Intuition

Walk into an established and well-reputed crystal store, and do nothing but look around initially. Walk around the store and identify if you feel any kind of emotional or visual attraction toward any particular crystal. The exercise takes a bit of time, and therefore, you must be patient with yourself. If you don't connect with any crystal for the first time, go back and return the next day.

Typically, if you are looking at a set of crystals, and you feel drawn toward one of them, then it is usually a vibrational match for your energy frequency. Take your eyes away from the stone that you feel an initial attraction for and, after some time, look at it again, and see how you feel.

Hover your dominant hand over the crystal or better still, hold it in your hand. Close your eyes and observe any subtle energy changes or vibrations you feel in your body. If you do, then this crystal is definitely calling for your needs. You can go ahead and choose it.

Remember that you may not always be able to discern the subtle vibrational changes in energy when you hold the crystal, especially as a beginner. In such cases, go ahead and make your choice based on your initial reaction. Use the crystal for a week or two, and observe your experiences. With patient practice you will find it increasingly easy to discern energy changes regardless of how subtle they are.

So, regardless of what you want the crystal for, trust your gut instinct and play along with it. And one of the most valuable suggestions you can get is to not overthink excessively about your choice of crystals.

In fact, you don't need to study and research the different types of crystals available before making your choice. Choose what attracts you, and then do a bit of research. More often than not, you will see that your choice of crystal matches with your needs.

Another piece of useful advice you can use is to take things slowly. First, take one crystal, use it for a week, and see how you feel and connect with its auric energy. Observe and make notes of the behavioral and attitudinal changes in your life, in yourself as well as those of others around. The changes are likely to be very subtle, and, therefore, you must focus a little more than normal to observe.

Once you are fine with what is happening, then you can go back and choose more crystals for yourself.

Finding the Right Crystal in a Virtual Online Store Using Your Intuition

Nearly all virtual stores will have some basic information and pictures of the crystals for you to choose from. Look at one page of pictures, and see which one attracts you the most or on which of the crystals do your eyes linger.

Most often, the crystals you are attracted to in a particular situation is relevant in your life for that time. Instead of trying to find 'scientific and logical' reasons for your attraction, know and believe that your intuition is telling you what your soul needs. Which is why, it is important to trust your intuitive powers and go along with its calling.

Until now, you are focusing on the crystals you are drawn to. You can shift your perspective for a moment, and focus on those crystals and gemstones that you feel repelled against. Those are the ones that you must definitely avoid choosing at that point in time because your intuition is telling you that the vibrational energy of that crystal is not aligned to your present needs.

Receiving a Crystal as a Gift

Sometimes, people can choose crystals for you, and when this happens, remember that the crystal has chosen to be with you even without you stepping out to make your choice. The stone has literally found a way into your life through a caring friend. If you receive a crystal as a gift, then accept it wholeheartedly with an open mind in the same way you accepted your initial attraction to a stone when you went shopping for your own crystal.

However, receiving crystals as gifts usually comes at a later stage in your crystal collection journey. As you increasingly connect with crystals and through them to the universal power, your needs and desires are caught onto by the universe, and using the law of attraction, the universe finds a way to get your crystals delivered to your doorstep. Typically, such deep desires to have a particular crystal to achieve a particular purpose are realized in the form of gifts.

Taking this point in the reverse direction, suppose you lose a crystal. Yes, you will feel bad about losing it, and you could shed a few tears and be disappointed in yourself for being careless and not looking after your beloved stone well. However, you must remember that it is very likely that the stone has served its purpose in your life, and the universe has found a way to pass on the benefits of its power to someone else that needs it. So, just like how crystals find their way to you when you need them, they could go away from you when their purpose is served. Therefore, learn to let go if you lose anything in your life.

Choosing a Crystal Based on Its Properties

If you are looking for a crystal for a particular ailment or problem, then you can find gemstones that are known to help in solving these problems. For example, there are specific crystals like aventurine that has a vibrational energy suitable to boost confidence. So, if you are looking to build confidence, then you can choose an aventurine. The next two chapters are a beginner's guide on the most popular crystals along with their healing powers and properties.

In fact, aventurine is not the only stone that helps to boost confidence. Even crystals like bloodstone, carnelian, etc. are great for this problem. You can go through all the crystals based on a specific property you are looking at, and then make your choice from among these using your intuition's guide.

Finding the Right Crystal Using the Pendulum Dowsing Method

Using the pendulum dowsing method is a bit of an advanced technique, and requires you to have a bit of experience. Yet, even for a beginner, it makes sense to know how it works. Use the following steps for this method:

Find the right dowsing pendulum - Think about what kind of dowsing pendulum you would like to have. There are numerous crystal-based pendulums you can choose from, and also you can make a simple one at home too. An easy-to-make do-it-yourself dowsing pendulum needs a tea bag or a favorite bead or a favorite crystal or stone tied to the end of a string.

Cleanse and clear the pendulum of negative energies - If you already have a pendulum that you use for your divination purpose, then you might already know how to cleanse and clear your instrument. Otherwise, you can use the same process employed for cleansing and clearing a crystal for the pendulum too. Chapter Four in this book deals about crystal care in detail.

Connect with and build a lasting relationship with your pendulum - You have to learn the language of the pendulum and connect with it to build a lasting relationship with your divination instrument. This step is important so that you understand and catch the messages that you pendulum is trying to tell you every time you use it for divination purpose including choosing the right crystal. Follow these steps to connect with your pendulum:

• Take a few deep breaths and ground yourself

• Seek support and help from the universe to help you achieve your purpose. You can use your own prayers or ask in simple language for help.

• Ask some basic questions to your pendulum to understand yes, no, or maybe answers it might choose to give.

For this to work, remember to ask questions to which you already know the answers. Other ways of setting up a communication channel with your pendulum include:

Ask your pendulum, 'what is a yes?' and wait for the answer. It could move clockwise or counterclockwise. Make a note of this reply.

Next, ask your pendulum, 'What is a no?' or 'What is maybe?' and wait for the answers, and make suitable notes.

- Another way you can establish a communication channel with your pendulum is by getting responses to questions like:

Am I male or female?

Is it right that I am [fill in your age] old?

Are my eyes brown?

Do I enjoy reading?

The yes/no answers given by your pendulum will help you know how your pendulum is connecting with you.

Now, your pendulum is ready for use. Place your chosen crystal on a table and hold your pendulum over it. Watch for the signs given by your divination instrument and make your choice of whether you want to take this crystal or not. Your divination pendulum is a great tool to help you make many choices.

Other Elements of the Crystal to Focus On

While being guided by your feelings and intuition is the best way to choose your crystals, here are some more elements you should focus on while making your choice:

Form of the crystal - Typically, most crystals emit their power through the edges, and the most intense power comes from their tips. The form of the crystal you choose depends on its use. A stone that has multiple edges and splintered tips will radiate and emit its energy through all the edges and tips. However, the energy radiation may not be uniform when you use these forms.

Spheres, on the other hand, radiate their energy uniformly. However, the radiation from a spherical-shaped crystal will be weaker than when emitted through an edge. Usually, crystals that are cut to a specific shape tend to have more radiation power while tumbled stones tend to radiate energy more gently, softly, and harmoniously than other forms.

Quality of the crystal - Stones that display the unique characteristics of a particular crystal are of better quality than those that don't display the expected traits. For example, the quality of a clear quartz is determined by its brightness. The more cloudy it is, the lesser the quality of the clear quartz.

On the other hand, a transparent ruby is more powerful than an opaque one. And yet, you must remember that the looks and profile of a stone is less important than its potential power. Follow your gut feeling here too, and even if you feel a stone is not what it appears, but your intuition powers are on a high when you hold it, then the crystal could be right for you. Remember that sometimes crystals simply need cleansing and cleaning to regain their original luster.

Size of the crystal - The larger the size of the crystal, the more power it can radiate. A small-sized amethyst will radiate power only to a short range of distance whereas a big druse or collection of amethyst crystals can radiate power to cover an entire room. Therefore, you must choose the size of your crystal based on your needs.

For example, if you want to place a stone so that it radiates its power to clear the negative energies from a big room, then you must choose a large-sized crystal or maybe even a cluster of crystals. However, if you want to wear a crystal around your neck, then you can choose a small one because the contact of the stone with your skin will enhance absorption by your body.

Most experienced crystal healers believe in gentle and slow healing rather than a blasting effect. Make your choices sensibly and prudently based on the above three factors.

Other Tips While Choosing Your Crystal

Here are some more tips you can use while choosing your crystal.

Avoid making your choice when you are feeling mentally or emotionally imbalanced - For example, if you are tired, stressed out, angry, or even excessively happy, don't go shopping for crystals. It is likely that wrong ideas find their way into your head based on the emotions you are experiencing.

Don't choose crystals for others - In fact, as a beginner, completely avoid choosing crystals and gemstones for other people, including your loved ones and close friends. Remember that choosing a crystal has to do with matching an individual's energy vibration with that of the gemstone.

You will not be able to read and decipher someone else's energy vibrations during the initial phases of crystal healing lessons. Even if someone gives you permission to choose crystals for them, it takes a lot of study and practice, and only the top scholars in the realm can confidently do this work accurately. It is best to keep crystal healing and choosing methods to make choices for yourself alone.

Approach this exercise with an open mind - If you have chosen to access the power of crystals, then it means you are ready to take the plunge without over-analyzing things excessively. If you are looking for 'scientific and logical' proof of every action and thought, you are unlikely to find success. In fact, these doubts will color your choice and you are bound to make mistakes. Therefore, it is imperative that you approach the exercise of choosing the right crystal with an open mind, and trust your intuition to guide you.

Finally, sometimes, despite your best efforts at trying to find a suitable crystal, you realize that you are not drawn to any of the stones that you have come across until now. You don't have to worry about it. Maybe, the time is not yet right for you to connect with the crystals that are shown to you by the universe through any channel.

If nothing attracts you powerfully, then accept the fact that the time is not yet right for you. Wait and keep your desires alive, and you will find your stone sooner rather than later. Another point of warning is to beware of buying crystals to simply hoard in your house. You run the risk of having stones with energy vibrations unsuitable and even harmful for your life.

Holding onto crystals without any purpose or meaning will reduce this exercise to a mere hobby, and crystal healing is more than a hobby. It is a calling. So, listen to your intuition and follow its guiding light. You will never be led astray by your own intuition. Believe in its power and take a leap forward.

And, of course, when you go on your crystal-finding journey, remember to expect the unexpected. You could go in search of finding lost love, and you could end up finding your true love, and realize that the love you lost had a greater purpose than you thought.

Chapter 9: How Crystals And Chakras Relate For Your Wellbeing

We have already seen how the seven chakras are categorized, and their specific locations in the tangible body. Let us now analyze the way specific harmonizing crystals help in the whole healing process.

Muladhara or Chakra One

This one is associated with the crystals Hematite; Black Obsidian; Black Tourmaline; Red Zincite; Garnet; and Smoky Quartz. They all help to stabilize your system and keep you grounded. They also enhance your physical energy; your willpower and your feeling of security. Of course, you do remember that this chakra is located at the lower end of your spine. So, even physically, taking care of this part of your body also helps in enhancing the focus of the relevant energies. The colors associated with Chakra One are red and black.

Svadhisthana or Chakra Two

The crystals associated with this chakra include Orange Calcite; Vanadinite; Carnelian; Blue-green; Turquoise; Fluorite. What they do is enhance your desire; your sexuality; and your creativity. Likewise, they keep your intuition at its peak. They also contribute greatly in your emotional and physical healing. Remember physically this chakra is located just below your navel. The colors associated with Chakra Two are orange and blue-green.

Manipura or Chakra Three

This chakra is associated with Citrine; Yellow Jasper; and Golden Calcite. It facilitates and enhances your intellect; ambition; and personal power. It also makes you feel protected. Of course, you remember that this chakra's location is just below the breastbone. Yellow is the color associated with Chakra Three.

Anahata or Chakra Four

This chakra that is located around the heart does well with the crystals Rose Quartz; Pink or Rubellite Tourmaline; Watermelon Tourmaline; Green Aventurine; Malachite; and Jade. What these crystals do is enhance love and compassion. They also enhance your emotional balance as well as global consciousness. The colors associated with Chakra Four are pink and green.

Vishuddha or Chakra Five

This chakra that is located just above the collarbone is associated with the crystals Sodalite; Blue Calcite; Blue Kyanite; Angelite and Blue Turquoise. Its representative color is blue. It helps you express yourself eloquently and provides you with divine guidance. Suffice it to say, Chakra Five is your center of communication.

Ajna or Chakra Six

The crystals associated with this chakra include Lapis Lazuli; Azurite; and Sugilite.

This chakra whose location is between your eyebrows is linked to the color, Indigo. It enhances your spiritual consciousness; psychic power; intuition; and light.

Sahaswara or Chakra Seven

Chakra 7, which is located at the head crown, is associated with the crystals Amethyst; White Calcite; and White Topaz. It is in charge of your energy; your consciousness of the world; enlightenment and a sense of perfection. It is linked to colors Violet and Golden White.

To be at peace with yourself, the environment and other people as well, you need to learn to use the healing crystals and their corresponding colors according to their different strengths and point of convergence. When you master this natural healing process, your energies will flow optimally, hence keeping your body in sync with your mind and spirit. You will find yourself with a very healthy balance and a contented feeling of wellbeing.

Chapter 10: How To Start A Crystal Colllection

Choosing a Crystal for Yourself

Make sure you are well educated on each of the crystals you collect. The best way to choose a crystal is to feel its energy. Trust your intuition and your sense of what feels right to you. Let yourself be guided to the crystal, so let it choose you.

There is a wide range of experiences that crystal shoppers report when choosing a crystal. Often, I personally feel a good vibe and a slight tingling sensation.

- Heat emitting from stone
- A dash of light from the crystal
- Cold energy
- Lightheaded sensation
- Ringing Ears
- A sudden rush of excitement

You should also take note of crystals that you feel you dislike. More often then not they represent qualities or issues you need to deal with.

Choose By Crystal System

Each crystal is part of a different crystal system with specific properties. The crystal systems include:

Hexagonal crystals, which manifest

Isometric crystals, which improve situations and amplify energies

Monoclinic crystals, which protect and safeguard

Orthorhombic crystals, which cleanse, clear, unblock, and release

Tetragonal crystals, which contain or ward off energies

Amorphous "crystals," which have differing properties.

Choosing By Color

The importance of color extends far beyond personal preference. Each color has its own vibrational energies with associated healing properties. By choosing a crystal of the crystal system that has the properties you'd like it to display along with the healing principles of the color, you can select crystals quite specifically for certain conditions.

Choose By How They Make You Feel

When you choose a crystal, you should hold it in your hand and see how it makes you feel. Note whether or not they make you feel comfortable or uncomfortable if they feel heavy or light, and if you feel other sensations. You should feel a pleasant feeling.

Pairing Crystals

Like wine and cheese, some crystals pair well to make them better than the sum of their parts. Crystals that pair well have complementary energies that can really help focus energy. For example, the energy of any crystal is amplified when paired with clear quartz. Here are some other pairings that work well:

Smoky Quartz and Apache Tears – a powerful combination for people who are grieving.

Amethyst and Labradorite – can help you get a more restful nights' sleep.

Citrine and Black Tourmaline – can help ground you in prosperity.

Rose Quartz and Ruby or Garnet – excellent for pairing relationships

Black Tourmaline and Clear Quartz – help facilitate the free flow of balanced energy.

Choose By Using a Dowsing Rod

considered to be a more advanced process, but beginners can effectively learn how to use one in order to discover the best stones for their initial practice. Keep in mind though that pendulum dowsing might require a higher level of intuition.

As one of the oldest forms of divination, pendulum dowsing allows us to discover the energy of crystals, guiding us towards the one that is most attuned to our spirit. Of course in the process of finding a pendulum, it is important that you find the right one for you to help guarantee a seamless and effective experience.

To choose a pendulum, observe a selection of them. Your spirit will know what is best for you and will gravitate you towards the right one without you having to exert any cognitive effort. Once you have a pendulum, you can start using it to choose crystals, ask it questions, or it can assist you in making decisions that result in a yes or no answer.

Steps in using a pendulum dowser for crystal selection:

Clear your mind – before starting any of kind of process with crystals, it's important that your mind is clear from possible distractions. Take a few minutes to focus on your breathing and set your mind to the goal of the dowsing experience.

Practice Your Pendulum

Different pendulums vibrate with different intensity and quality. So what feels like a 'yes' with one pendulum, might feel completely different from another. To attune to your specific pendulum, hold it in your hand and close your eyes. Ask it a question to which you know the answer will be yes. Once you've felt the vibrations of a yes answer, ask it a question whose answer would be no. you should be able to sense a change in the vibration of your pendulum. In doing this, you develop a deeper sense of your pendulum, thus allowing you to better understand where it wants to guide you.

Choose your crystals – When using a pendulum dowser to select crystals, simply hold the pendulum over the crystal, or over an image of the crystal if you're buying it online, and ask it a question referring to the crystal. Try not to make suggestions in your mind to influence the answer of the pendulum as this could interfere with its true recommending. Try to maintain an open mind.

Where to Shop

There are many sources where you can purchase stones –both in brick-and-mortar stores and online. Many towns and cities have retail crystal outlets. These may be listed as metaphysical bookshops, crystal stores, or New Age shops. With knowledgeable staff, most will let you handle the crystals before you purchase. You can also find traveling mineral or gem shows are a great place to purchase crystals and can't be beaten for selection or price. Although these usually need to be planned for in advance. You can even buy crystals online when making a purchase ensure that you're working with a reliable seller. You may want to use your pendulum when ordering crystals online.

Crystal Starter Kit

Clear Quartz – if you don't know which crystal to use, start with clear quartz; it works with every type of energy.

Smoky Quartz – is the crystals a lot of people use because it's a manifestation stone that converts negative energy into positive.

Citrine – promotes self-esteem and prosperity

Rose Quartz – supports all types of love, including unconditional and romantic love.

Amethyst – helps you tune into intuition and guidance from higher realms, as well as the power of your dreams

Black Tourmaline – is a grounding stone that is protective and that keeps negativity at bay.

Rainbow Fluorite – deepens intuition, promotes love, and facilitates clear communication.

Carnelian – helps you set appropriate boundaries, have integrity and be creative.

Hematite – is protective, grounding, and centering and can also attract energies you'd like into your life.

Turquoise – promotes good luck, prosperity, and personal power.

Sacred Geometry of Cut Stones

You can find crystals cut into many different shapes, including spheres and polyhedrons, which have varying properties. Working with stones cut into these shapes will impart the properties of both the crystal and the sacred shape.

Dodecahedron – the dodecahedron is associated with the element of the Ethereal realm and connects you to intuition and higher realms.

Hexahedron – the hexahedron, or cube, represents the element of earth. It is grounding and stable.

Icosahedron – the icosahedron is linked to the element of water. It connects you to change and flow.

Merkaba – the Merkaba is a 3-D star. It contains all five of the above polyhedrons within it and therefore combines all the effects of each. It is also associated with the energy of sacred truth and eternal wisdom.

Octahedron – the octahedron represents the element of Air and promotes compassion, kindness, forgiveness, and love.

Sphere – the sphere has the energy of completeness, wholeness, and oneness.

Tetrahedron – associated with the element of fire, a tetrahedron promotes balance, stability, and the ability to create change.

Other Names for Crystals

In recent years, some retailers have given brand names to crystals and have in some cases marked them. The reason they are typically branded is usually that it originates from a particular area on property owned by the people who brand it, but the location does not greatly affect the properties of the crystal.

- Amazon Jade is Amazonite.

- Aqua Terra Jasper is either resin or onyx.

- Atlantis Stone is Larimar.

- Azeztulite is and has the same properties as clear quartz.

- Boji Stones can also be found non-branded as Kansas pop rocks.

- Healerite is generically found as Chrysolite.

- Isis Calcite is the branded form of white calcite.

- Lemurian Light Crystals are a branded form of Lemurian quartz.

- Mani Stone is black-and-white jasper.

- Master Shamanite is the same as black calcite.

- Merkabite Calcite is white Calcite

- Revelation Stone is brown or red jasper.

- Sauralite Azeztuline is quartz from New Zealand.

- Zultanite is the mineral diaspore.

- Agape Crystals are a combination of seven different crystals: clear quartz, smoky quartz, rusticated quarts, amethyst, goethite, lepidocrocite, and cacoxenite.

Crystal Safety

In general, working with crystals is relatively safe. However, some crystals contain substances (such as aluminum, copper, sulfur, fluorine, strontium, or asbestos) that are toxic to humans, so do not put them in the bathtub or make a crystal elixir with them. It's also best to wash your hands when you've finished holding them. These crystals include:

- Aquamarine (contains aluminum)
- Black Tourmaline (contains aluminum)
- Celestite (contains strontium)
- Cinnabar (contains mercury)
- Dioptase (contains copper)
- Emerald (contains aluminum)
- Fluorite (contains fluorine)
- Garnet (contains aluminum)
- Iolite (contains aluminum)
- Jade (contains asbestos)
- Kansas pop rocks (contains aluminum)
- Labradorite (contains aluminum)
- Lapis lazuli (contains pyrite, which contains sulfur)
- Malachite (contains copper)
- Moldavite (contains aluminum)
- Moonstone (contains aluminum)
- Prehnite (contains aluminum)

- Ruby (contains aluminum)
- Sapphire (contains aluminum)
- Sodalite (contains aluminum)
- Spinel (contains aluminum)
- Sugilite (contains aluminum)
- Sulfur (contains poisonous)
- Tanzanite (contains aluminum)
- Tigers eye, unpolished (contains asbestos)
- Topaz (contains aluminum)
- Tourmaline (contains aluminum)
- Turquoise (contains aluminum)
- Zircon (contains zirconium)

Now that you understand the fundamentals of crystals and chakras and how they work, we can go on to applying this information with crystal grids. To put it simply, a crystal grid is a method of working with crystals that involves creating very specific arrangements of different geometric shapes or patterns. These patterns usually include some type of sacred geometry in their form.

When used properly, these grids can amplify the power of the crystals even more. While it is possible to get good results from the use of a single crystal, when you use a grid, it can only enhance the results and give its energy a significant boost.

To create your own crystal grid, you first need to establish a foundation or a base to work with. The shape you use can be printed on a piece of fabric or a paper. Some have engraved wooden boards that they can lay out to place their crystals on. In some cases, you can even obtain a template to show you exactly where to place your crystals for the best effect.

Why You Need Them

You can use a crystal grid for many different reasons. Some people use them primarily for spiritual connections, but they can also be used for healing, to provide protection, to find love, to achieve prosperity, or any other number of things.

When you use the crystal grid, the collection of crystals all working together has an increased power that works alongside the sacred geometry to harness extra energy to work on your behalf. They also serve as a solid anchor when you need them.

As you can probably imagine, there are many ways to create a crystal grid, each with its own unique benefits to you. While there may be many reasons to justify using a grid, we can break them down into four different categories.

Crystal Energy: Because of their unique structure, crystals work really well when used in certain patterns. The crystal grid helps to harness even more of their properties to give you added support in accomplishing your goal.

It is important to choose those crystals that have the very properties you're searching for. To achieve your intended purpose, you may have to think beyond the obvious though. If for example, you are looking to improve your chances of success, then you would obviously choose crystals that will help you to achieve that goal, but you could also include crystals with related properties like determination, prosperity, and self-confidence to support it. Together, the power of all of these elements can help to direct their energy in the right direction for you.

Sacred Geometry: There is a form of metaphysical science that supports the belief that certain patterns that are found in nature are actually a fingerprint for understanding the universe and how everything in it actually works. These shapes are referred to as sacred geometry and they represent the actual framework of all creation.

Each of these shapes has its own use and form of energy. While not every crystal grid uses sacred geometry, when it does, it makes the entire grid far more powerful than one that does not. When using sacred geometry, choose your grids very carefully to ensure that the power you will receive will be directed towards your actual purpose.

Using sacred geometry also is beneficial in helping you to transmit your energies out of the grid into the rest of the universe so that the results can be manifested. You can also channel that energy inward to heal your broken aura to improve yourself when needed. The point is that while crystals have their own unique powers that can help you, using them with specific chakras within a grid can enhance their power even more. If you use a crystal grid with sacred geometry, you get the most intense power possible in the metaphysical world.

Numerology: Crystal grids used with the ancient spiritual science of numerology is very similar to sacred geometry. By selecting the number of crystals based on their symbolic meaning and energy as it relates to the grid, you can connect to support your purpose and better connect to their energy. Not only does this amplify the energy emanating from them, but it channels it better to focus on a very specific task.

Your Intention: Don't forget the power and the energy that is generated by your own thoughts. When you can transmit that information to crystals, especially when they have been carefully placed on a grid, this is when they really work their best. You can program your crystals with your thoughts and dreams. The grid will store them and broadcast them out into the universe for as long as you need them to.

These grids can become powerful tools in your hands and are extremely effective.

However, in order for you to get the best results, you must follow through on any intentions you transmit to them. Their power is a source of energy and motivation, but you will not receive rewards for anything that you don't wish to work on. They can only connect to something that is real within you and broadcast that intention around the clock for as long as you need them to in order to effect the change that you need.

Chapter 11: How To Choose Your Crystal?

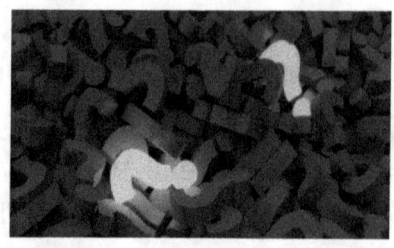

To choose your crystal, you need to know about crystals and personal zodiac sign. Throughout history, people have been using zodiac stones whether keeping in their home or using it personally. But in today's world, these stones have been replaced with birthstones. There is nothing wrong with it, but using zodiac stones are more appropriate in this case because they have more vibrational energy rather than using birthstones which have less and are gemstones. Zodiac stones have more reach to your planet per your zodiac sign and it has more power to support your need, depending upon the kind of stone you use. Of course, it will be in regards to your zodiac sign so that you can amplify your positive characteristics, simultaneously, balancing the negative characteristics. Here are the lists of stones with their zodiac signs:

Aries: Blue Tiger's eye, Unakite, Fire Agate, Citrine, Emerald, Bloodstone, Carnelian, Aquamarine, Apache Tears, Aventurine, Amethyst, Clear Quartz, Diamond, and Smoky Quartz.

Taurus: Pink Calcite, Onyx, Malachite, Green Aventurine, Amber, Copper, Rutilated Quartz, Selenite, Rose Quartz, Lapis Lazuli, Rhodonite, Emerald, Jape, Blue Tourmaline, and Pink Opal.

Cancer: Selenite, Rose Quartz, Ruby, Rhodonite, Red Jasper, Leopardskin Jasper, Moonstone, Citrine, Emerald, Carnelian, Fire Agate, and Sunstone.

Leo: Sunstone, Ruby, Pietersite, Mahogany Obsidian, Peridot, Garnet, Amber, Pyrite,

Tiger's eye, Howlite, Labradorite, Onyx, Carnelian, Citrine, Amethyst, Yellow Jasper, and Heliodor.

Virgo: Sugilite, Sapphire, Snowflake Obsidian, Charoite, Tree Agate, Carnelian, Mookite Jasper, Moss Agate, Chrysocolla, Howlite, Green Aventurine, Amazonite, Amethyst, Hematite, Magnetite, and Sapphire.

Libra: Morganite, Moonstone, Mohagany Obsidian, Blue Lace Agate, Blue Tourmaline, Lapis Lazuli, Citrine, Jade, Ametrine, Apatite, Bloodstone, Sapphire, Opal, Pink Tourmaline, Tiger's eyes, and Boulder Opal.

Scorpio: Sodalite, Smoky Quartz, Rhodochrosite, Natural Citrine, Red Jasper, Labradorite, Aquamarine, Black Tourmaline, Amethyst, Black Moonstone, and Yellow Topaz.

Sagittarius: Labradorite, Blue Lace Agate, Lepidolite, Amethyst, Imperial Topaz, Sodalite, Turquoise, Snowflake Obsidian,

Smoky Quartz, Lapis Lazuli, Peridot, Blue Goldstone, Blue Topaz, Black Obsidian, and Jet.

Capricorn: Ruby, Emerald, Rainbow Obsidian, Smokey Quartz, Red Tiger's Eye, Onyx, Jet, Malachite, Fluorite, Garnet, Black Tourmaline, and Amber.

Aquarius: Larimar, Moonstone, Rainforest Jasper, Garnet, Hematite, Apatite, Aquamarine, Amethyst, Amber, and Angelite.

Pisces: Black Tourmaline, Iolite, Turquoise, Ruby in Kyanite, Labradorite, Lapis Lazuli, Fluorite, Jade, Bloodstone, Blue Lace Agate, Amethyst, Blue Quartz, and Aquamarine.

To use your stone, you need to know what sort of crystals or stones come into your horoscope and then decide from which stone you want to start your journey with. The implementation can be depended on what your internal body demands. Whether it wants to heal faster from some disease, or whether it wants to get rid of the negative vibrational energies inside it, or both—it's your call. It is better that you spend your time with crystals in a personal space so that you have access to the universal energy source surrounding yourself. You can recharge with it, or you can rejuvenate. Your personal space where you use your stone can help you in overall development and can provide you with the needed strength to overcome whatever you are looking for. Experiment with each stone. See how they suit you. Trials and errors are a must in life, so work yourself with each stone and see what benefits the most.

The more you touch your stone, the more you utilize its energy. To wear your crystals, you can wear it as jewellery, or as regular beauty products. You can even use them as your purse or can place it under your pockets. The other way you can wear your crystal is to start your day with a crystal layout. For instance, you can place

Fluorite to your third eye chakra and Amethyst over your heart chakra. If you place these crystals for five minutes before going out to your job, then you will feel an energy shift within you. You can try this with different crystals per your horoscope. You can even use the crystals with your meditation. With meditation, you can attain your true self, your inner peace. You can dive deeper into your consciousness and can understand the level of your spiritual being. A source for transformation, meditation is best for mind, body, and spirit. Holding different crystals, not at once, but learning to use them at different time, and also not praying to them, is an effective way to enhance your ability to reach a place of quiet stillness. To enhance your abilities with crystals and meditation is to be first comfortable. You don't have to sit in a lotus position. You just have to feel comfortable. Just breath in and breath out. Putting your attention on breathing will allow you to access the oldest methods of meditation techniques. Be consistent in your meditation. Try using a particular stone for a week or a month and find out thorough tests what your stone is.

To choose your stone can be the question of choosing the right stone for someone you want to present it as a gift. To do that, you need to listen to what your heart is saying. You might be giving crystals to someone for personal growth, healing purposes, or the development of intuition, or it can be any reason. Listen to what your heart says and see which stone you are getting attracted to that you want to give someone. Find that inner knowing. Other ways to choose the right stone to give might depend on the crystal's properties. You might be giving the stone in a gesture that your friendship may get repaired, or the same thing can be said about loving relationships. Knowing the properties of the stone can help you to decide which direction you want to go.

You can narrow down your choice with this, shortlisting crystals based on their properties. Or your choice to give the right stone to give to someone might be random. In this case, you have to trust the universe. You might not have any specific choice or the influence of what you should give. Simply spread the various crystals in front of you, or if you are in a crystal shop, in either manifestation, close your eyes. Take a deep breath. Then ask the universe to show you the way to guide you for the highest stone.

You can even combine crystals with crystal therapy. The therapist will recommend to you different sessions depending on your experience with crystals and your progression. Also, depending upon your health, the session will help you to experience detoxification of negative energies. This can help you to discover the underlying surface of your thoughts. The therapist will use different crystals in regards to how the different crystals correspond to your body, also, helping you to decide your crystal in the absence of the therapist when you have to work alone with the crystals.

Other ways to choose your crystal is to understand the dynamic between crystals and their colour. Scientifically, colours has been linked to affecting human being's emotions and moods. Understanding how the colours of the crystals influence its vibrational energy, you will be able to select crystals based on their healing abilities, how you can balance chakra centres, and create a life toward a more positive journey. For instance, if you are getting irritated by colour then it means that you need to work on something to improve your life. If you getting attracted, for example, by the colour pink, then it means that it is the right time for a new beginning. Other meaning could be that you are empathetic and you need support. You are showing compassion toward somebody. For your emotions to be kept at balance, you need somebody. With the way you see colours and react, you can choose your crystal. The colours of the crystals have their influence on its properties. Below are the colours of crystals and what those colours depict:

Gray: Astral travel, open-mindedness, dream recall, balance, and dream work.

Black: Shadow-side work, change, self-reflection, protection, and personal growth.

Brown: Nature spirits, inner peace, grounding, stability, and shielding.

Teal: Tranquillity, harmony, inner peace, spirit guides compassion, and portals to angels.

White: Meditation, protection, purification, divine connection, and sacredness.

Pink: Inner-child work, friendship, compassion, empathy, and new beginnings.

Violet: Personal growth, ascension, transformation, conscious awareness, and spirituality.

Blue: Justice, wisdom, authenticity, communication, self-expression, truth, and integrity.

Indigo: mental expansion, psychic awareness, intuition, and spiritual growth.

Yellow: Mental clarity, self-confidence, inner strength, courage, willpower, and bravery.

Green: Prosperity, emotional healing, love, physical health, abundance, and compassion, growth.

Red: Instinct, motivation, passion, physical healing, vitality, protection, and stability.

Orange: inner-parts work, creativity, emotional balance, transformation, sexuality.

You can work with a particular colour at a time to choose the right crystal for you because a different colour indicates its efficiency for specific conditions. Again, trial and error can help you decide what colours to choose and how to heal yourself through positive vibrational frequencies, while eliminating the negative ones, working to achieve the balance of mind, body, and soul.

Chapter 12: Overview On Visualization

Representation expects you to need something, see it, and trust in it. After some time, when you are working toward a path towards your objective, the procedure and vitality you put into perception will start to move your life a positive way.

Perception expects you to need something, see it, and have confidence in it. After some time, when you are working toward a path towards your objective, the procedure and vitality you put into perception will start to move your life a positive way.

While perception sets aside effort to ace, there are a few different ways to begin profiting by its influences right away.

Picture yourself opening the icebox. Picture yourself taking out a lemon. Hold the lemon in your palms. Feel the surface of it's waxy, yellow strip and its smoothness, and feel the yellow strip finishing at a point. Marginally press the lemon in your palm, and feel the nearness of new squeeze inside. Take a sharp blade and cut the lemon in two parts. Naturally discharged particles of the lemon scent hit your nose. Smell the lemon scent. Presently nibble into the lemon.

In the event that your mouth has salivated at this point, you simply had an incredible representation experience. You haven't really chomped into the lemon, yet your mouth salivated as a general rule. That is the intensity of representation.

Representation is an exceptionally incredible method for accomplishment of achievement throughout everyday life. Representation basically implies realization of something at the top of the priority list, however that thing may not exist in all actuality. Perception isn't something enchantment. Representation for progress is a system to be performed dependent on discoveries landed at by specialists after research. It is outstanding that competitors and sportsmen are educated to rehearse procedures of perception for pinnacle execution.

It is currently entrenched by specialists in the field that each creation which you see around yourself was a thought first. Everything, for example, the structures, the vehicles, the streets, the furnishings, the pen, the paper, the PC, was first envisioned by somebody in quite a while mind. Each creation, including you and me, has its cause as a top priority. God first envisioned us in quite a while mind and have made us in His very own picture.

To prevail in any undertaking, along these lines, wouldn't it be consistent to initially imagine your achievement in your inner consciousness? Surely it is. Give me a chance to reveal to you how.

I have been rehearsing this perception procedure in my life since long. At the point when I was another legal advisor, I regularly used to envision myself standing unquestionably in the court, before judges, on my feet, and contend out my customer's case in the most influential way.

Perception systems have helped me extraordinarily in my prosperity as a legal counselor. I keep on rehearsing this representation system even at this point. With my eyes shut and keeping in mind that hitting the sack, I actually find in my inner being, the court in the entirety of its subtleties; the Honorable judges sitting on the dais; I hear my case being gotten out by the Court Reader; me strolling unquestionably and moving toward the Bar; and starting my contention discourse in a sure style; confronting the court inquiries in a balanced way and keeping up my balance all through and still, at the end of the day barraged with troublesome inquiries; fulfilling the court and influencing them in my mind; the way of my articulation; the tone of discourse; my signals and so on.

You can apply this perception strategy to prevail in any part of your life. You may improve connections, for example, dating the most alluring young lady, having superb association with your life partner. You might have the option to become familiar with the new abilities, for example, open talking, driving a vehicle. You can even figure out how to be progressively sure and self-assured utilizing representation system, for example, moving toward the manager for a raise/advancement, disapproving of something that you would prefer not to do. You also can rehearse representation for making progress in any part of your life.

• Identify a mind-blowing aspect which you need to prevail in.

- Practice perception consistently while hitting the hay and each morning on arousing.

- Close your eyes and make mental pictures during perception.

- Let your psychological pictures be in however much detail as could reasonably be expected.

- Have the perception experience through your very own eyes. This implies you need to envision as though you're in reality. You ought not take a gander at yourself from a third individual's perspective.

- See yourself really prevailing in your undertaking during your perception procedure.

- During representation experience, blend your feelings with the experience.

Accept, emphatically accept, that whatever you are envisioning WIIL show in all actuality. Keep in mind your perception experience isn't only the mind's play. You are really making, and submitting a request of your craving, aim with the universe.

To accomplish best outcomes, disguise the envisioned understanding. Give it a chance to turn into a piece of your being.

Understanding the mind's job in inspiration and conduct is one of the most basic components in physical wellness achievement. In the event that you battle with changing propensities and practices or on the off chance that you can't get roused, at that point even the best preparing and sustenance program is useless.

An entrancing reality about your non-cognizant personality is that it's totally deductive in nature. At the end of the day, it is completely fit for working in reverse from the conclusion to the methods. You don't have to have the methods or the "know how" to accomplish an objective at the time you previously set the objective, in such a case that you "program" just the result (the objective) effectively into your "psychological PC," at that point your subliminal will dominate and enable you to locate the vital data and means and do the activities important to arrive at your ideal end.

Numerous individuals know about confirmations and objective setting procedures as approaches to offer guidelines to your intuitive personality. In any case, maybe a definitive method to take advantage of the magnificent forces of your brain is to utilize the system called representation. In one regard, attestation and representation are one in the equivalent, since when you talk or think a certification first, that triggers a psychological picture, being as the human mind "thinks" in pictures.

You can utilize perception to program objectives into your intuitive personality. It's straightforward: You close your eyes, and rationally make pictures and run motion pictures of your ideal final products. For instance, you can envision your body, in as clear detail as could be allowed, precisely the manner in which you need it to look. Whenever rehashed reliably and inwardly, mental pictures are acknowledged by your intuitive as mandates to be done and this assists with evolving propensities, conduct and execution.

Advantages

Increment inspiration

Inspirational representation includes envisioning achieving your ultimate objective and the sentiments that go with that achievement. Invigorate every one of your faculties, and drench yourself in a psychological picture so a lot of that it shows up genuine to you. By acquainting yourself with sentiments of accomplishment, you increment your inspiration to arrive at your ultimate objective and accept achievement is increasingly conceivable and sensible.

Characterize what you need

Figure out how to remove your consideration from what you don't need, and spotlight on what you wish to involvement. Perception enables us to evacuate all the feeling encompassing cynicism, and rather, place our consideration on activities that will empower us to make individual progress. When you characterize your objective, keep on rehearsing representation consistently. The more nitty gritty your representation, the closer your objective will appear to you.

Increment positive considerations

For the duration of the day, we have a continuous inner exchange with ourselves. Become mindful of your contemplations, and pick them cautiously - you need to be a companion to yourself, not a damaging foe. By expanding positive contemplations today, you start to welcome positive results into your life. You won't start to see changes the principal day, yet fortification it is like planting a seed. Promptly, you will feel more joyful, and after some time, things will start to move in your life.

Advance execution

One sort of mental symbolism that builds our exhibition is to imagine yourself in high-weight circumstances. By rationally preparing for testing conditions, you can create adapting methodologies and better react to future tensions. Jim Bauman, Ph.D., the counseling sport therapist for USA Swimming says to name something near you that will remind you to keep up a solid point of view when times get flawed. For instance, the letter "P" on your PC can remind you to take a point of view that spotlights on your advantages, and not on negative musings.

Lessen pressure

Representation is perhaps the most ideal approaches to recover your brain on track when you feel out of parity. Tuning in to slow music and picturing your day sorts out your contemplations, rationally get ready you, and lessen pressure. Another pressure alleviation procedure - and my undisputed top choice - is to lie on your back and envision all the worry in your body is warm magma amassed at the highest point of your head. At that point, gradually envision it pouring down your ears, neck, shoulders, and whole body. You ought to really feel a sensation move down your body as you envision the pressure leaving your head. I utilize this to nod off, and I have never remained alert past my shoulders.

Inventive representation, implies making a picture or a scene or envisioning something in your brain, with eyes open or shut. That picture or scene or creative mind, is then used to supplant any torment or adapt to any misfortune, by appending positive emotions to it. However, innovative representation isn't just about managing torment or misfortune. It likewise helps support confidence, improve states of mind, battling tension and so on.

Our brain can envision some truly interesting things. These things don't should be genuine or even bode well. In the event that it is believable, our mind will envision it. The intensity of innovative perception lies in its capacity to influence our mental, physiological and social conduct.

The cerebrum is equipped for making two sorts of pictures. Give us a chance to see them in detail:

1. Visual Imagery

This type of inventive representation is the place a picture can be seen, voices can be heard and now and again you may even feel the impacts. Most imaginative perception includes visual symbolism.

Ordinarily when we envision a sea shore or some type of water, we find in our brains a delightful shore, the sound of the sea and in the event that you are an incredible innovative one, you even feel the sand underneath your feet!

2. Non-Visual Imagery

This is when there is no image development in the psyche. In any case, every single other sense together help one envision. So when a prepared performer tunes his instruments or attempts to recollect a music piece, it is non-visual symbolism which becomes possibly the most important factor. He can hear the sound or feel the strings of the instrument and judge if everything is in order or not.

Innovative perception has an incredibly solid effect on individuals. The manner in which we think, respond, act, and so on can be adjusted with the assistance of innovative perception. Give us now a chance to take a gander at the advantages of inventive representation.

As a matter of first importance, the advantages of innovative representation are felt in all circles of life. It is generally utilized in medicines and different circumstances where these sorts of imaginative perceptions prove to be useful.

• Therapeutic Benefits

If there should be an occurrence of different mental issue, an individual is dependent upon inventive perception. In the event that an individual is experiencing nervousness issue, they are approached to imagine tranquil, quiet and calming scenes. The hints of the ocean are played and they are approached to quiet down, envisioning a coastline. This causes them quiet down, without utilizing any medicine.

At the point when an individual is experiencing physical agony, they are approached to picture easy and wonderful things, while the other drug produces results. This is done on the grounds that when in torment, consistent consideration regarding the agony exacerbates it appear than it really is.

• Forgetting Fear

Regularly individuals suffer from sudden anxiety at the absolute a minute ago. This is characteristic, yet it turns into an obstruction to their exhibition. Be it in front of an audience, in a test corridor or anyplace. To deal with such a circumstance, one can envision post triumph scenes. This causes us to get over a minute ago nerves and put forth a strong effort.

• Morale Booster

From time to time, our spirit goes down. We feel low and not propelled enough to complete things. Through inventive perception we can persuade our psyche to envision all the greatness and prizes that anticipate us toward the finish of the action. This causes us get up and at any rate start.

A similar representation likewise causes us complete assignments once we start them.

• Mood sponsor

Normally, on the off chance that we are ending up progressively certain, diminishing pressure and encountering more delight then our disposition will be sure also. At the point when we dream of each one of those things that satisfy us, we consequently put into movement, the procedure of overlooking our issues.

Phases of Creative Visualization

1. Picture Generation

Here the picture appears. We start envisioning and framing a psychological picture, here and there from memory, now and again from dream and at times from both.

2. Picture Maintenance

Here we attempt to keep the picture alive. Our psyche is inclined to overlooking effectively. Thus, this progression is tied in with keeping up and keeping the picture alive in our brains, long enough to really consider it to be genuine.

3. Picture Inspection

Presently, our brain might be absent minded, however it has an incredible consideration for detail. So the subsequent stage includes a careful assessment of the picture to cause it to appear as genuine as could be allowed. This includes contrasting the picture with other mental pictures and our genuine encounters.

(No doubt... the brain really does all that. Also, here we thought just we perform multiple tasks!)

4. Picture Transformation

This is the last and most significant advance. Making it genuine. The picture which was just piece of the psyche, is currently experienced by the brain and body the same. The impacts of the symbolism, be it alleviating, quieting, calming, and so forth are altogether felt and appreciated in the last advance.

Imaginative perception is substantially more troublesome than we give our mind kudos for. It can frequently be a depleting knowledge, physically and inwardly. In any case, when we do it, when we accomplish innovative perception, we are regularly left with a feeling of profound quiet and quietness. Issues appear to settle themselves and we are left feeling loose.

Conclusion

Thank you again for purchasing this book!

I hope this book was able to help you to understand and appreciate the healing and stress-relieving effects of crystals.

The next step would be to decide which crystals are most appropriate for you and your intentions. Then, utilize the knowledge learned from this book so that you can finally achieve internal balance, maintain a stress-free existence, and reach the optimum state of wellbeing that you deserve.

www.ingramcontent.com/pod-product-compliance
Lightning Source LLC
Chambersburg PA
CBHW070100120526
44589CB00033B/1097